THE SIMPLE

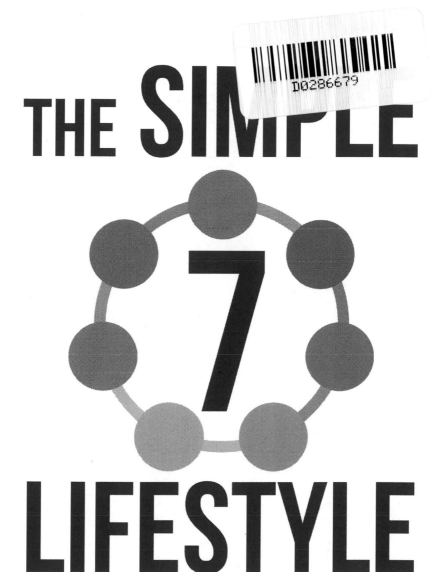

7

LIFESTYLE

YOUR ROADMAP TO GET HEALTHY, STAY HEALTHY, AND LIVE YOUR BEST LIFE!

JERALD DUGGAR DC, FDN-P
TAMMIE DUGGAR CTNC, CCNE

Live Well!—
Be Well!!
♡ Dr Jerry
+Tammie

First Edition: October 2021

Printed in the United States of America

ISBN: 9798485816001

Interior design by FormattedBooks

CONTENTS

ACKNOWLEDGEMENTS

To our parents who have given so much of themselves to make our lives what they are today. We've learned from your successes and your setbacks, and you have taught us to be resilient in the face of challenges. You've taught us to trust in the Divine Purposes of life and your love for us has given us the confidence to dare to dream big and to pursue our passions.

PREFACE

DR. JERRY'S STORY

I can still clearly recall the day. I was flying home back to my home in Georgia where I was attending chiropractic school after being in Utah to attend my father's funeral.

He had been in poor health since I was a young boy. When I was about 12 years old, I remember my mother rushing outside to tell me that my father had suffered a massive heart attack while he was at work.

I remember standing on the sidewalk as my mother raced to the hospital. I was confused. I thought heart attacks only happened to really old people and my dad was in his early 50's. It was scary to think that I might not ever see my dad alive again.

We were fortunate; thanks to modern medicine, my dad miraculously survived that massive heart attack. It had taken a team of surgeons to perform a quadruple bypass surgery to get the blood flowing back to normal.

My teen years were marked by the memory of a father that was barely able to work, who took dozens of medications, and complained about some aspect of his health all the time. When he finally passed away, he had about 10 diagnosed chronic degenerative conditions. It was heartbreaking to witness.

Unfortunately, my dad didn't know any better. His doctor never taught him about healthy lifestyle habits. Never challenged him to give up his cola habit. Never told him that most of his diseases were self-induced. Instead, he'd go to the doctor with a complaint, and he'd come home with a prescription for another drug.

As I sat on that plane to return to Georgia, I pondered his life. I recalled his health habits: his "addiction" to Coca-Cola, his lack of exercise, his overall diet loaded with sugar, his inability to manage emotional stress, and his negative outlook on life. It was obvious why he never felt well and why the doctors couldn't help.

There was a much better way, and I knew it.

You see, just a few months earlier, I had suffered my own health crisis. The stress of full-time chiropractic school, two part-time jobs, and volunteering at my church on Sunday had caused me to disregard my own health.

I was losing weight, my skin was a mess, I couldn't sleep, my gut was bloated, and I was depressed. I even had a momentary complete loss of my ability to manage my anger and nearly severely injured my young child. There I was, devoting my life and future career to becoming a doctor, someone who would advise others how to live their lives better, and my own life and health were falling apart. It was a sobering wake-up call.

At my wife's insistence, I reached out to my nutrition professor, Dr. Paul Goldberg, DC, an early pioneer in natural and functional medicine. He quickly helped me get to the root of my problems. Over the next several months, my wife and I worked to reset our priorities and our habits to rebuild my health foundation. We quickly addressed the myriad of food sensitivities I had developed. We tried to take more time to be mindful and intentional about our entire lives. I lowered the intensity of internal pressures that I was placing on myself with school, and I tried to reduce my work demands.

What I witnessed was a profound and rapid restoration of health and happiness. It didn't happen overnight, but it unfolded in the natural timing of my body. The process became another testament to me of the power of my body to heal.

As I sat on that plane, I saw how natural, lifestyle-based medicine quickly solved the same sorts of problems that caused my father to suffer needlessly for decades.

I committed to myself and my future patients that I would be the kind of doctor who was willing to have the hard conversation. I was going to be the kind of doctor who would constantly teach, by example and precept, that the solutions to our health problems lie in the way we live our lives every day. I was going to teach my community that we are either creating health or disease with every decision we make.

It's that passion and commitment that lies at the heart of this book. I care about helping as many people as I can to get a hold of their health by working on the key areas of their lifestyle. The "Simple 7 Lifestyle" model can be made so simple that you can easily adopt these behaviors into your life.

Imagine yourself in 12 weeks with more energy, a clearer head, better sleep, clearer skin, and improved hormone balance. It's not only possible; it's almost inevitable if you can create better habits in the seven key areas of your life that we'll cover in this book.

TAMMIE'S STORY

I got off to a rocky start in life. I was born six weeks premature and only weighed 3 pounds 11 ounces. The doctor discouraged breast-feeding because I was so small, so I missed out on what we now know is a critical time to develop a healthy gut and immune system.

Consequently, as a small child, I always had digestive issues and allergies. My seasonal allergies lasted most of the year. I was sensitive to animal dander, perfumes, and fragrances; even raw fruits and veggies would often cause my mouth to itch and my throat to feel like it was closing off. It seemed like I was continually battling sinus infections and strep throat. I was constantly bloated and gassy, which led to some painful nicknames and lots of teasing from my brothers.

Because my mom was a nurse for a pediatrician, I received just about every medication in an effort to find something that would work to treat my symptoms. My symptoms never really went away, but as I got older, I learned to live with them, thinking I'd deal with these issues all my life.

In 1992, Jerry and I started seeing a local chiropractor and learned about natural healing. Much to my surprise, after a few short weeks of getting chiropractic adjustments and implementing his suggestions to improve our lifestyle, my seasonal allergies went away! I witnessed firsthand how my body could heal when I changed my habits and rebalanced my nerve system and this made me fall in love with natural healing. That's why I was so excited when Jerry realized that he wanted to be a chiropractor. Before long, we were driving our moving van across the country to Georgia for his chiropractic education.

As Jerry mentioned in his story above, while we were in chiropractic school, Jerry's health meltdown was a rude awakening for both of us. When his lab tests came back and his doctor explained that many of his problems were related to what he was eating, I realized that I needed to be an active partner in helping him to get better. That testing changed our world forever! I can still remember sinking to the kitchen floor, crying from feeling overwhelmed.

I had always taken great pride in my skills in the kitchen. I was a good cook, but I didn't know anything about cooking gluten and dairy-free. I was completely knocked off my foundation and didn't know where to begin.

My prayers were answered when a new friend from church took me under her wing and opened me to the world of nutritious food. Although it was sometimes challenging, my friend helped me learn to adapt my favorite recipes with new ingredients. My kitchen became my playground, a sanctuary for creation. The most important thing I realized is that nutritious and delicious food options are abundant.

Once liberated from the boring sameness of the Standard American Diet, I became a self-proclaimed "real-foodie." Together, Jerry and I made significant shifts in our entire approach to eating. While he kept plugged into the latest research on the role of diet on overall health, I worked on perfecting the implementation of what he was learning.

We tried just about all the popular diet approaches of that time: juicing, vegetarianism, food combining, anti-candida diets, alkaline diets, and more. Along the way, we paid careful attention to what worked to restore our health and help us feel our best. We learned essential principles in each "system" we experienced.

We noticed a big difference in our overall health. As the years went on, though, I noticed that my tummy troubles from my childhood gradually returned. By 2009, I often found myself doubled over from excruciating pain in my abdomen for hours at a time.

This was such a frustrating experience because I thought I was already eating great! After a thorough workup, we were able to understand the full picture of what was going on. I learned that I had developed an overgrowth of bacteria in my small intestine called SIBO (which stands for small intestinal bacterial overgrowth). That diagnosis answered so many of the lingering issues I had experienced throughout my life.

Clearing SIBO and balancing my gut was not an easy task. It took close to two years. I had to be patient. When my test results finally came back negative, it was such a happy day! Now my digestive symptoms are few and far between, and I finally feel better than I have for decades.

I often reflect on all the incredible things I've learned along my journey. I needed to follow my body's healing timeline. I know how frustrating it is to want a quick fix, but the body doesn't work like that; it heals layer upon layer.

My own life experiences inspired me to take my love of cooking and blend it with my passion for nutrition, which led me to become a Certified Culinary Nutrition Expert. I was able to add hundreds of hours of research on the most current diet and gut healing approaches to my decades of "in the trenches" personal experience. Through my challenges, I have mastered both practical and straightforward real-life solutions.

My journey has also helped me understand so many of my client's emotional challenges as well. I felt my heart leading me to work with other people who are frustrated and may feel lost and confused, so I devoted a year to becoming a Transformational Nutrition Coach through the Institute for Transformational Nutrition.

I love the opportunity of sitting knee-to-knee (or computer screen-to-computer screen) with people who are dealing with health issues that are a bit scary and overwhelming to them. My heart is filled with so much empathy and love because I've been where they are now. My heart is full of hope and confidence because I know they can make a difference in their health. They can heal and feel amazing in their body! I understand that the answers they are looking for are available. If they are open and trust in timing, they will find their answers.

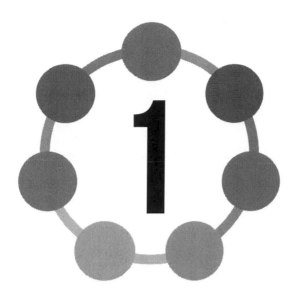

THE BIG "WHY"

THE TSUNAMI OF CHRONIC DISEASE

Most of us are painfully aware that we're not as healthy as we'd like to be. Our lives feel chaotic and out of balance. As a society, we eat more and more food but get less value from it. Our internal and external environments have become more and more toxic. We're overstressed and undernourished.

America now ranks 37th in overall health and 38th in life expectancy. Over 130,000,000 people suffer from chronic diseases that science reveals are 78% preventable. The number of people diagnosed with chronic diseases has quadrupled in the last 40 years. 65% of Americans are overweight or obese, and obesity is related to over 300,000 deaths each year. The price tag to manage this skyrocketing problem of chronic disease is estimated at more than 2.7 trillion dollars. If the trends continue, economists expect that by 2082, it will take the entire Gross Domestic Product to pay for this growing crisis.

Unfortunately, there's a trend in the medical world that only makes matters worse. Too often, patients receive treatments that won't actually help and can even be dangerous at times.

A story published in *The Atlantic* describes a man seeking treatment for his coronary artery disease. Two doctors recommended he receive a coronary angiogram, "in which a catheter is threaded into an artery to the heart and injects a dye that then shows up on special x-rays that look for blockages. If the test found a blockage, the cardiologist advised, the executive should get a stent, a metal tube that slips into the artery and forces it open." The man wanted to find out more and learned that instead of the procedure that had been recommended for him, over-the-counter medication was actually recommended as the first step for relief.

After learning more, the man was fortunate enough to consult with Dr. David L. Brown, who is part of the Right Care Alliance, a group on a mission to stop the trend of "increasing medical costs without increasing patient benefits." Through Dr. Brown's guidance, the patient avoided getting a stent and instead worked on improving his diet and started medication. Within three months, "his cholesterol had improved markedly, he had lost 15 pounds, and the chest pain never returned."[1]

This type of situation is far too common. Our society's current approach to our health crisis is unsustainable. So, what should we do? Is there any real hope for our health to improve? If so, what does it take to transform?

Our current model waits until a person is already in the heavy grasp of chronic disease symptoms before making improvements. How do we shift away from this damaging practice? How do we address the underlying causes of the problem that are almost always rooted in a person's daily lifestyle?

These questions are what has motivated us to create the **Simple 7 Lifestyle**™. This wellness approach may not completely change

---

[1]   https://www.theatlantic.com/health/archive/2017/02/when-evidence-says-no-but-doctors-say-yes/517368/

our entire nation's health overnight, but we know that it can change the trajectory of every person who embraces it. That's why we're so excited you're starting here; you're taking the first step to change, the first step to a more balanced, healthier lifestyle.

What you have in your hands is a simple framework with proven clinical results. We'll focus on the big picture principles that have stood the test of time and form the foundation for a lifetime of health and happiness. We're going to help you take control of your body and your health.

Close your eyes for a minute. Picture yourself with more energy, more vitality, and down to your ideal weight. Can you see it? Can you feel it? How awesome is it to see yourself in that state? Won't it be fantastic to get there? To look and feel better than you ever have before?

We are excited about your journey of self-discovery, healing, and rebirth. You will face physical and emotional obstacles along this journey but remember that you are not alone!

SKILLS BEFORE PILLS

The entire Western world has been seemingly seduced by the giant medical complex that has been promising good health in the next drug, potion, or pill over the past century. Better living through chemistry has been the rallying cry. To most doctors, hospital administrators, and policymakers, the thought that the first line of defense against degenerative disease could be as simple as lifestyle change can't even get a seat at the discussion table.

Of course, we need heroic, life-saving medications and invasive surgery. Still, we've become intoxicated with the idea that we can abuse the laws of health for years, and then when we're suffering from disease, our doctors will give us a chemical to trick our body into thinking it is healthy. On the surface, most people recognize how absurd this notion is, yet we aren't provided any other consistent and workable alternative path to health. As a society, we continue to follow the path of least resistance and abdicate our responsibility to the medical establishment.

Even the "alternative" health movement has been mostly unsuccessful in helping people develop the skills and behaviors that lead to real wellness. Instead of addressing the habits that remedy our deficiencies, too many people jump right to taking a handful of vitamins, herbs, and natural treatments. There is no way for supplements to make up for a terrible lifestyle!

The key to achieving long term results is to develop a balanced lifestyle to support the way our bodies are designed to work. Don't wait for a magic pill or procedure to fix you when it might be too late. Follow our framework to give yourself a fighting chance against degenerative disease and the opportunity to live with an abundance of health and energy.

THE SIMPLE 7 LIFESTYLE

What are the key elements to this lifestyle, and how do we apply it daily? Consider this your first official coaching session as we summarize the habits that make up the Simple 7 Lifestyle. Over the next seven chapters, we take a deep dive into these key daily practices, but we'll briefly introduce them to you here.

STRATEGY #1: THINK WELL
The ability to engage in productive, positive, and purposeful thoughts about self, others, and life in general with a clear vision for the future.

Most of us carry around a fair amount of negative baggage that creeps into our thoughts every day. We pick up patterns of thinking and beliefs about ourselves early on in life, and often these patterns continue to play out in our minds for years or even decades. In many ways, we can only outgrow our limited beliefs about ourselves when we learn to recognize them and critically evaluate them.

We'll discuss how we can create a more intentional and meaningful life when we start with a clear vision of what we want to help create in the world. We will then focus on controlling our thoughts and becoming more mindful and present.

"Thinking well" means becoming a conscious creator and being positive and optimistic about our life and our future.

STRATEGY #2: SLEEP WELL
The ability to consistently restore and revitalize our health each night with restful sleep.

Sleep is one of the most overlooked aspects of a healthy lifestyle. The average adult needs 7-9 hours of quality sleep every night to repair and heal. Unfortunately, many aspects of modern living have sabotaged our sleep/wake cycles, and the number of people with some level of insomnia continues to grow.

We'll offer powerful tips and solutions to help you get the rest your body is quietly craving.

STRATEGY #3: BREATHE WELL
The ability to properly and efficiently give our body the most essential nutrient of all: oxygen.

Breathing is so essential for life that it might seem that there is really nothing to it. Why would we need to focus on how to do it "better"? Well, it turns out that there really is a right and wrong way to breathe. We'll show you how to turn the simple act of breathing into a powerful health practice.

STRATEGY #4: EAT WELL
The discipline of creating a diet based on clean, real, and nutritionally dense food and pure, clean water, even in a world that seems to be so confused about what to eat.

There may not be a more contentious topic in the health world than that of diet and nutrition. There are dozens of competing camps, each with smart-sounding scientists claiming that following their eating code is best for humanity. Instead of promoting that one approach is better than all the rest, we'll teach you to tailor your dietary choices to your specific needs based on your health status (or disease status, as the case may be).

We'll introduce you to the concepts of "ancestral nutrition" or what others call a "paleo template" as an appropriate foundation to build your own personal ideal diet.

In addition to a nutrient dense diet, it's best to drink clean, pure water and reduce or eliminate our intake of soda, coffee, milk, fruit juices, and energy drinks.

STRATEGY #5: MOVE WELL
The ability to naturally move our bodies through their full range of motion with ease and add specific and appropriate exercise to create an active lifestyle.

The modern lifestyle has become more sedentary than in the past. We sit more and move our bodies less. Research proves that even those who exercise an hour every day can lose the benefits from that exercise if they remain sedentary for the rest of the day. We'll share our simple ideas of how to create a foundation of movement and activity every day. We'll also explain why we advocate High-Intensity Interval Training (HIIT), bodyweight-based exercises, and yoga to build strength, stamina, and flexibility.

STRATEGY #6: LOVE WELL
The ability to create and nurture relationships with self, family, friends, and associates that lift, inspire, and add joy to life.

As the famous Dean Martin song so clearly states, "You are nobody until somebody loves you...so find somebody to love." Without connection, intimacy, friendship, and the knowledge that we are important in others' lives, we can't feel lasting happiness. Humans are social creatures who need connection and love in order to thrive.

In what can often be a cruel twist, developing and maintaining deep and lasting relationships is one of the hardest things to do. Other people let us down and frustrate us. Other people don't always do what we want them to do. We often take for granted those people who are closest to us. Taking time every day to nurture your most important relationships is vital to wellness because, as Dean Martin continues, "You may be king. You may possess the world and its gold. But gold won't buy you happiness when you're growing old."

 STRATEGY #7: PLAY WELL
The discipline to take enough time for recreation, plea-sure, and enjoyment of all life has to offer.

The powerful strategy of play is often lost as we grow into adults. We forget all the great things we learned through having fun, being creative, and playing games as kids. In addition to being a power-ful stress reducer, time spent in "play energy" activates parts of the brain that are often neglected and helps us function more wholly as human beings.

Making time for recreation, fun, and play daily balances our body, mind, and spirit. Time spent playing, whether playing a sport, a board game, or even writing and creating, is not time wasted! It is a powerful aspect of wellness.

HOW TO USE THIS BOOK

Our goal isn't to overwhelm you. We certainly don't expect you to master all aspects of the Simple 7 Lifestyle strategies at once. That would feel like you're trying to juggle 7 balls simultaneously. Take this process as slow as you need to. The positive changes in your life will unfold steadily and naturally over time.

You might be asking, "But where do I start?" Great question. The answer depends on your current lifestyle. We'd recommend that you complete a simple self-evaluation to find your weakest area and focus on that first. As you improve in that area, you can shift attention to the next habit in line.

TAKE ACTION: THE WELLNESS WHEEL

Our first activity, The Wellness Wheel, will help you determine where you stand in each of the seven categories. Completing this exercise will give you direction on where to focus as you begin your health journey. Follow these steps:

1. Each spoke on the Wellness Wheel represents one of the 7 Simple Strategies. Mark a dot on each spoke to rank your progress for that particular habit. The closer you are to the center of the wheel, the more you need to work on that area. The farther from the center, the better that habit is in your life. Don't overanalyze each point; just make a mark based on your first reaction.
2. Connect each dot (like a dot-to-dot) around the wheel.

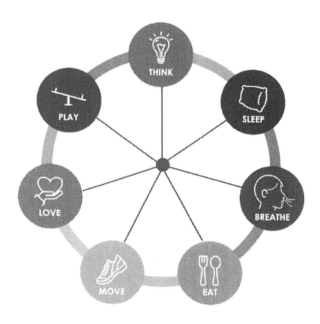

THE EVALUATION AND ACTION PLAN

Is your Wellness Wheel a smooth circle, or is it a bit bumpy? Think about that for a minute. If this were an actual wheel, how efficiently would you move? Wouldn't it be nice if you could make some adjustments so the road to wellness is a smoother ride?

Now that you've plotted out your current situation, it's time to set goals. Find the point closest to the center, which should represent your least developed habit, and make goals to improve this area and plan to implement these goals in your daily life.

When you've made improvements in that area and have established a new habit, move to the next point on your wheel. You won't make massive changes overnight. It might take several weeks or even months to establish these new habits, and that's okay. While you're concentrating on creating new habits in a particular area, keep up with the others you've already established. You worked hard to strengthen your weaknesses!

We recommend you do this self-evaluation every few months to track your progress and recognize the areas where you're struggling.

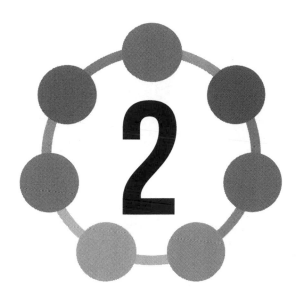

THE JOURNEY

SUMMITING THE PEAK

You've probably heard the famous Taoist saying that a journey of a thousand miles begins with the first step. Each of us is on a healing journey, and we don't know how long or how difficult the road ahead of us will be. How many twists, turns, and obstacles will we encounter along the way?

In the summer of 2009, I (Jerry) had a memorable experience that taught me to keep going, even when we don't have the perfect vision of what's to come. I got to accompany a group of Boy Scouts to Pfeifferhorn Peak, one of Utah's tallest peaks that overlooks the Salt Lake Valley at 11,331 feet. There's no easy route to the summit. All approaches require a trek of at least 4.5 miles and over 3,700 ft of elevation gain.

In good weather, hikers can make it to the summit and back in one day, but the other Boy Scout leaders and I planned an overnight campout for the boys. There were two beautiful glacier-fed lakes about halfway up the mountain where we could make camp and do a little fishing. We all threw on our 30-pound backpacks and headed up the trail. We had an experienced leader in the front, another leader in the middle of the pack, and I brought the rear to make sure we didn't lose anybody.

I thought I was in good shape, but I was surprised at how quickly the hike became strenuous and how much more difficult it was carrying an extra 30 pounds. Before long, I was panting while brooding over the uncomfortable shoulder straps on my backpack. I was also secretly grateful for the few scouts whose slower pace allowed me to take my time and enjoy the scenery. The dense vegetation along the trail made it so there was no visible sight of the peak we were to climb the next morning.

After about 3 miles of hiking, the terrain flattened out a bit, the trees cleared, and we could see the lake where we would camp for the night. From that vantage point, I saw a broad mountain peak just to the south of the lake and assumed that was the Pfeifferhorn.

After we set up camp, the boys fished and played around for a while, and then we cooked a simple dinner and tried to persuade them to get some sleep.

We quickly broke camp in the morning and each packed only a small daypack before heading off. Once again, we made significant elevation gains in just a matter of minutes, but this time with less weight on our backs and a relatively good night's sleep. We all found the hike much easier than the day before. Within a short time, we made it out of the tree line and onto a rocky ridge leading up toward the peak we'd seen from our campsite.

The peak I had assumed would be our ultimate destination was called the "false summit," and we still had a long way to go. Once we reached the top of this point, we could see a beautiful trail leading through boulder fields and a ¼ mile-long knife-edge ridge to the second steep climb to the true summit.

The last 200 yards were the toughest of the whole climb. It wasn't a straight shot to the top; we had to scramble up the side of the summit. Once we all made it and were standing on the windy peak, overlooking the beautiful landscape as far as we could see, we felt that all the hard work had paid off. The view was breathtaking, and each of the boys felt a sense of accomplishment. We learned powerful lessons that day about perseverance, hard work, focusing on a goal, teamwork, and the value of preparation.

THE IMPORTANCE OF VISION

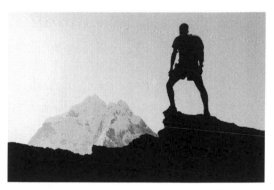

I witnessed one of the most amazing views I've ever seen as I stood on that peak. The sky was clear; I could see hundreds of miles in every direction. I could see the path I had taken to get to the summit. I could see cities in the distance below and several other famous mountain peaks along the Wasatch range.

What if I had stopped at the first "false" peak, thinking, "Hey, this is good enough,"? I would have missed out on that incomparable view and the sense of accomplishment that comes from finishing something difficult. What if I had started that hike without a goal in mind at all? I probably wouldn't have made it too far since that first day of the hike was more challenging than I had anticipated.

The first step along your journey to health is to capture a vision of how you want your life to look. You must know where you're going and why you want to get there. You may not know exactly how incredible it will feel, just as I didn't realize how majestic that mountain view would be, but you can visualize the things you want: a body that functions as it should, days, weeks, and months with more energy, better sleep, and improved relationships. What do you want your life to look like? Imagine feeling the best you *possibly* can.

We don't always have a clear vision; it gets clouded every day due to the complexity of our world. However, you can have clarity on your powerful purpose. Yes, you'll run into tough terrain. There may be moments when you feel like you're carrying too much extra weight. Maybe you'll even want to stop when you're just part way there but grasping that ultimate vision will keep you on the right track.

"You cannot stay on the summit forever; you have to come down again. So why bother in the first place? Just this: What is above knows what is below, but what is below does not know what is above. One climbs, one sees. One descends, one sees no longer, but one has seen. There is an art of conducting oneself in the lower regions by the memory of what one saw higher up. When one can no longer see, one can at least still know."

—Rene Daumal

THE CONSCIOUS CREATOR

Many of us have become slaves to our programming. We're accustomed to waiting for the world to change around us, and we respond and react to our external stimuli. What would your life look like if you took control and responsibility for all results and outcomes that affected you? We've asked ourselves this question throughout our own healing journey, and it's a question we ask all our clients.

You can shock yourself into new behaviors that create temporary results, but real improvement and change can only happen by developing new habits. Henry David Thoreau penned the phrase, "Things do not change; we change." The changes you choose to make will shift how you express health and live your life.

So, what's the secret to making lasting change? We may want immediate transformations, but creating new habits comes down to setting goals and sticking with them. Without a goal, there is nothing to work for. Without the commitment to that goal, you'll never achieve it. When you connect to your powerful purpose, your reason for being, there is no obstacle you can't overcome.

The biggest hurdle on the way to your big goals is most often hopelessness. When you've been sick, tired, in pain, or just not feeling like yourself for so long, you may forget that it's even possible to feel good again. When you can't envision a better future than your present, making massive changes and commitments to new ideas can seem overwhelming.

We want to help you overcome that obstacle right now! By completing the following exercise, you will be able to connect to your powerful purpose and by doing so will have the strength to commit to the new habits that will create positive changes.

VISION EXERCISE: POWERFUL PURPOSE

It's tempting to skip to the parts of the book that tell you what steps to take for change, but in our experience, our clients who have the most long-lasting health improvements are those who take small actions with intention, purpose, and clarity. This exercise can turbo-charge your results and arm you with the mental toughness to overcome the inevitable obstacles along the way.

Grab your favorite notebook or journal. Find your favorite pen. Clear your schedule for 30 to 60 minutes and answer the questions below.

Section 1: The Effects of Your Current Health

1. What is the cost of feeling sick, tired, in pain, or just not feeling like yourself?
2. What activities have you been prevented from doing or what goals have you been prevented from achieving because of your current health situation?
3. What effect have these limitations had on you?
4. What effect has your sub-optimal health had on your relationships? Consider all of your relationships: spouse/partner,

children/grandchildren, friends/colleagues, and even your relationship with yourself.

Section 2: What is Your Vision?

1. What could you accomplish if your health was no longer an obstacle?
2. How would your relationships be different?
3. How would the quality of your daily experiences be different?
4. What would you do differently each day and how would that make you feel?

WRITE YOUR VISION LETTER

You've written about the challenges and limitations you've experienced because of sub-optimal health. You've also allowed yourself to imagine what your life could be like without those obstacles.

We have been through similar health challenges and have made it through to the other side. It's hard to make a total life change, but we know it's possible because we've done it. Our program is designed to help you reach big health goals, but your results will be up to you. *You* must put in the hard work.

Imagine what your life could be like in the next few months. Get specific and detailed about what you see. What does your life look like? How do you feel? What are your relationships like? What contributions are you making?

Find a place where you can be alone with your thoughts and write about what you envision for your future. You could begin your letter something like this: "Dear (your name), I can't believe the changes that have happened since I began my healing journey . . ."

Include the details about the many things you've experienced along your healing journey. Talk about creating new habits that have transformed your health. Write about your accomplishments and how you have grown. Envision how much better your relationships are with those you care about the most. Detail your feelings and emotions, how you look, and what you enjoy doing.

Write all the intricate details of what is happening in your life! Once you get started, let the words flow. Share every detail you can imagine. Write every word you want to express. Don't just sit and think—write it down! Writing these things will help you begin to create the changes you wish to see in your life.

Now, read your vision. Commit to doing everything it will take to accomplish or achieve what you described in your letter. Focus on the result, like "I commit to healing myself so that I can watch my grandchildren grow up." Or "I commit to a future where I have the energy to accomplish my goals." Commit to whatever inspires you. Print your commitment and place it in several places: your fridge, the bathroom mirror, your car, your computer. This will allow you to see your commitment several times every day and will help you stay motivated to work toward your ultimate goal.

"Until one is committed, there is hesitancy, the chance to draw back. Concerning all acts of initiative (and creation), there is one elementary truth, the ignorance of which kills countless ideas and splendid plans: that the moment one definitely commits oneself, then Providence moves too. All sorts of things occur to help one that would never otherwise have occurred. A whole stream of events issues from the decision, raising in one's favor all manner of unforeseen incidents and meetings and material assistance, which no man could have dreamed would have come his way. Whatever you can do, or dream you can do, begin it. Boldness has genius, power, and magic in it. Begin it now."

—William Hutchinson Murray

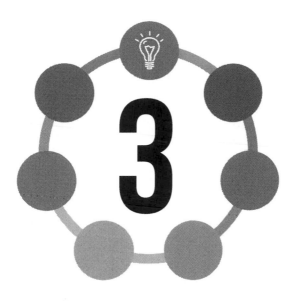

THINK WELL

MINDFULNESS

Has this ever happened to you? You jump in your car to run an errand and you arrive at your destination without any real recollection of any details of the drive? It's almost as if your brain wasn't even paying any attention to the thousands of little decisions involved in driving and you arrived there on autopilot. Sadly, we live too much of our lives on autopilot, especially when trying to get through the daily grind while also dealing with health issues. Instead of embracing life, the goal becomes: "Just make it through the day."

This is no way to live life—with or without health problems. When you discover your health isn't optimal, it's the perfect time to learn how to be more mindful every moment of every day.

Mindfulness is one of our favorite ways to manage stress continually. It occurs when you are simply in the present moment, without thoughts, judgments, or worries about the past or future. You truly experience what is happening right now with all five senses. We live most of our lives with some of our senses muted, but mindfulness reawakens the senses, bringing new meaning and purpose to life!

In the case of autoimmune disease or other health complications, mindfulness can be particularly rewarding. Let's say you are currently suffering from Rheumatoid Arthritis joint pain. You may have a habit of letting your thoughts race to the future, thinking things like, "My joints will one day be deformed." Using a mindful approach, you make nonjudgmental, compassionate observations about your body and the world around you as you are experiencing it right now.

People often find that these observations somehow decrease pain and suffering. Instead of ruminating on suffering, your focus is directed outward to the world around you.

The next time you find yourself thinking about the past or worrying over the future, try implementing these steps:

1. Take a deep breath and focus on your breathing.
2. After you have steadied your breath, engage your hearing. What do you hear around you? Is it pleasant or not? Do not make judgments like "bad" or "good," just calmly engage the sense of hearing.
3. Repeat step number 2 for all five senses.
4. Find yourself in the world around you. What are you doing? Where are you? How do you relate to what you saw, heard, etc.?

After you've grounded yourself in your surroundings, you will be able to engage more fully in the present moment, which is truly powerful and even life changing.

Without a conscious awareness of our internal and external worlds, we are quickly swept up into a life that is moving too fast, is too complicated, and too hard to control. The inevitable result is a busy mind filled with anxiety, worry, and stress. We must take some conscious action to manage stress better.

Since there is no way to magically remove all stress from your life, we all must concentrate our efforts on learning techniques that work for our circumstances and personality. We'll share some of our favorite stress management techniques that are proven to help reduce anxiety.

OVERCOMING NEGATIVE THOUGHTS

Your brain is powerful, but sometimes you need to keep that power under control. You may have thoughts that don't serve you; maybe you haven't even noticed negative thoughts that come to your mind, but nevertheless, they can hurt you.

You likely have a lot more negative thoughts than you realize. A group of business students was asked to maintain a record of "their naturally occurring thoughts for a period of two weeks." The students were encouraged to be "brutally honest" with their thoughts. The study revealed that 60-70% of the average student's thoughts were negative, though the students expected that 60-75% of their thoughts would be positive.[2]

We are too often our own worst enemies. Our negative self-talk can lead to self-loathing, which can then turn into self-sabotaging behaviors. And when we allow these thoughts to ruminate within ourselves, they can also be projected on other people, affecting some of our most important relationships.

Social media has also had a surprising effect on many of us throughout the years. While it can be an excellent source for keeping in contact with old friends or family, studies have found that there is a "strong link between heavy social media and an increased risk for depression, anxiety, loneliness, self-harm, and even suicidal thoughts." The reasons for this may be feeling inadequate, isolated, left out, or even too self-absorbed.[3]

---

[2] https://www.psychologytoday.com/us/blog/sapient-nature/201310/how-negative-is-your-mental-chatter

[3] https://www.helpguide.org/articles/mental-health/social-media-and-mental-health.htm

The good news is that you can change the way you think. You don't get to choose where you were born or what genetics you inherited, but you can choose to focus on more positive aspects of life. It's not easy, but it is possible! We have a few tricks that can help you to flip your thoughts.

MENTAL JUDO

We use a two-step process to help clear up negative thoughts before they turn into negative emotions and negative behaviors.

The first tool is called Mental Judo. Judo is a modern-day martial art form originating in Japan. One of its central principles is the idea of maximum efficiency, minimum effort. The idea is that resisting a more powerful opponent will always eventually result in your defeat but if you can use your opponent's strength of attack against him it causes him to lose his balance. His power will be reduced, and you may defeat him.

It works similarly when it comes to our minds. It is almost impossible to just "stop" thinking a negative thought. But what if we were able to take that thought, throw it "off-balance" a bit and then use that thought to create a powerful new thought? We call this process "mental judo."

With Mental Judo, your negative thoughts are the opponent, and we're going to show you exactly how to defeat them.

STEP 1: THE GRIP & FLIP

Most of us aren't aware of our repetitive thought processes, so it's helpful to slow down and "listen" to the thoughts we are thinking.

To really get a good grip on your thoughts, we'd suggest that you get two small notebooks or journals. Differentiate these journals somehow because one will be for negative thoughts, and one will be for positive thoughts.

Keep both journals with you throughout the day. When a negative thought comes to your mind, write it down in your "negative thoughts" notebook. Some common negative thoughts might be like these:

- "You're not (or I'm not) good enough"
- "You're (I'm) so stupid"
- "You're (I'm) worthless"
- "Nobody likes you (me)"

It's interesting to note that some people's internal dialogue is in the first person, and others' dialogue is in the third person. In other words, some people are talking to themselves, and other people are listening to "another" person's voice in their head. For this exercise, write the words down exactly as you "hear" them.

Now that you have captured this thought, it's time to conquer it mentally.

Take your "positive thoughts" notebook and write down two statements that are the exact opposite of the negative thought. Here are some examples:

- I'm good enough, and I'm amazing
- I'm smart, and I'm talented
- I'm priceless, and I'm valuable

If the same negative thought keeps coming back, continue writing it down in your "negative journal" and keep thinking of new ways to flip it into a positive statement.

A word of caution: your "negative journal" is just for you; don't poison anyone else's mind by letting them read it. Keep it private and personal. On the other hand, keep your "positive journal" out where you can read it often. If someone else sees it, they will feel good by reading the words too!

STEP 2: THE VICTORY DECLARATIONS

The second part of the process is to take the positive statements and convert them into personal declarations.

Make a list of your top 5-10 statements from your Mental Judo journal and turn them into a powerful declaration or affirmation about yourself. A declaration is a statement that is a truth, even if you don't quite believe it yet.

Here are some examples:

- I am beautiful/handsome
- I am smart
- I am talented
- I am loved

Put this somewhere you can see it every morning. Read it out loud, saying each declaration like you mean it. This step might feel weird to do, but you'll feel better about yourself and your life if you do this each day. Say your declarations every day until you believe them and become them. When that happens, you know it's time for a new set of declarations.

FEEL AWESOME LIST

Life can be so amazing, yet so overwhelming and challenging at times. What do you do when you need to feel more awesome?

That may not be a question you've considered, especially when you feel less than awesome. When you're down in the dumps, you may find yourself wallowing in self-doubt, self-pity, and even self-loathing for longer than necessary. Instead of going down the rabbit hole of negative feelings and emotions, use our Feel Awesome List next time you feel the gloom rising.

We've created a list of things that have helped us eliminate the funky negative energy that creeps into life far too often. Use our ideas as inspiration, then brainstorm and create your own Feel Awesome List to have on hand.

- Dance party! Turn on your favorite music and just dance.
- Acknowledge your negative feelings. Write it down and explore why you're feeling the way you are.
- Take a relaxing bath.
- Go for a hike or a nature walk.
- Listen to an uplifting podcast, audiobook, talk, or sermon.
- Think of three things you're doing well and say them out loud.
- Create a meaningful connection with someone.
- Take time to pray or meditate.
- Get sweaty! Move your body and let the negativity out in your sweat.
- Create positive thoughts by reciting affirmations or a mantra.
- Laugh! Search *Dry Bar Comedy* on YouTube for some fun, clean humor.
- Write in a gratitude journal. Remember, what we focus on grows.
- Remind yourself that you have everything inside of you that you need to succeed.
- Stop and identify where the feelings are coming from, then examine your thoughts about them.
- Let yourself feel the emotions that are overcoming you. Allowing yourself to take this time with your feelings may help them disappear quicker.
- Remember who you are, who you were, and who you want to be.
- Get coached. Work with someone who can effectively help you work through your difficulties.
- Do something you're good at.
- Create something. It can be anything you enjoy creating, whether it's a craft, food, a story, or anything else that comes to mind.

- Talk with a friend.
- Reflect on encouraging words from friends, like thank you notes, texts, or emails.
- Send a note to someone. Ask yourself who you can reach out to and let them know you're thinking of them.

Remember that your mind is powerful. If you've become victim to pessimistic thoughts and negative emotions, progression will be thwarted. Use these tools we've mentioned to create a new way of thinking, a new way of viewing yourself, your life, and your health. You don't have to remain stuck in a bleak mindset. You can use your mind as a gift.

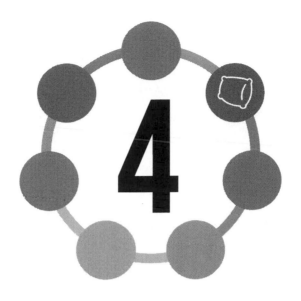

SLEEP WELL

TO SLEEP, PERCHANCE TO DREAM

Recently, we started helping a working mom that was dealing with insomnia. She was so exhausted from her lack of sleep that she blamed her lack of sleep for completely ruining her working life.

She'd done so well in her career that she'd received several promotions in the first six years, but when she had kids, her exhaustion skyrocketed. She couldn't concentrate, she could barely drive, and her mental health took a significant hit. This mother did what most people would do—reached out to her doctor, hoping to repair the damage insomnia had done to her life. Her doctors prescribed potent sleeping pills, but this woman knew that wasn't the right answer for her. She eventually left her job, attempting to work on her own, but felt that she missed out on a great deal of personal and professional development because of insomnia. She said, "I often dream of what my life could have been without insomnia."

Unfortunately, this story isn't all that uncommon. Too many people have dealt with feeling unsatisfied in their careers or even getting fired due to insomnia. Of course, it goes way beyond just the negative impact on the workplace. Sleeplessness can lead to anxiety and depression, along with other mental health issues.[4]

Sleep is one of our most precious resources, and we often undervalue its importance to our health, longevity, and quality of life. The health benefits of exercise will vary depending on how long you do it and the quality of your activity. Similarly, your sleep will benefit you more if it's for the right amount of time, and it is top quality rest.

Research has shown that sleep is just as critical as eating a nutritious diet when it comes to building a solid foundation for health. Sleep is just as impactful on our mental health as productively processing your emotions during or after stressful events, and it has been shown to be just as important as high-quality exercise for weight loss and fitness. Despite these facts, sleep tends to get overlooked when people embark on a health program.

Adults generally need between six and nine hours of sleep per night. Most adolescents and teens do best with at least nine hours a night, even though they think they can get by with four or five (remember bragging about how little sleep you got in high school and college?).

There are, of course, some exceptions. Some people can function well with less than six hours, and others need more than nine. One factor that can affect your sleep requirements might be a history of illness or emotional stress. Some people may need a lot more sleep during the winter months. Pregnant women require more sleep, especially during the first trimester.

If you feel tired when you first wake up, you probably aren't getting sufficient sleep. Observe how you feel immediately upon waking rather than after you're up and moving around. These first few moments of wakefulness before your mind fully kicks into gear

---

4   https://www.theguardian.com/careers/2017/jul/29/it-completely-destroyed-my-working-life-your-insomnia-stories

are probably the best measure of how your body is functioning and how your sleep is working.

THE PROBLEM WITH SLEEP DEPRIVATION

For most people who don't sleep well, sleep deprivation has become a pattern and not just an occasional night of restlessness. They can't recover quickly from a chronic lack of high-quality sleep. And unfortunately, you can't stockpile a supply to use later, nor can you pay your body's sleep debt back. You might feel rested and sharper after sleeping in, but the benefit is temporary and can be compared to depositing money in your account, then withdrawing it again a day or two later. Lost sleep is lost forever, and persistent lack of sleep has a cumulative effect when it comes to the havoc it can wreak on your health.

Many people often don't realize how detrimental sleep deprivation can be. Insomnia and sleeplessness are such a chronic condition that many don't even realize that they suffer from it. You might assume that the sleep you're getting is adequate if your eyes open when the alarm clock rings, and you feel reasonably alert once you're up and moving. If you've shorted yourself on hours and quality of sleep for too long, your state of sleep deprivation could feel normal to you. However, researchers tell us that a sleep deficit can have serious, far-reaching effects on a person's health.

A single night of sleeping only four to six hours has been shown to impact a person's ability to think clearly the next day. Studies have shown that good sleepers and poor sleepers experience about the same number of minor stressful events during the day, but good sleepers are less disturbed by them. Poor sleepers experience life events as being far more negative than those who sleep well.

Sleep deprivation can cause changes in brain activity similar to those experienced by people with psychiatric disorders. Sleep deprivation puts the body into a pre-diabetic state and can make us feel hungry even if we've already eaten. Interrupted sleep can dramatically weaken your immune system. Tumors grow two to three times faster in laboratory animals with severe sleep dysfunctions.

According to a new study led by a Harvard pediatrician, children ages 3 to 7 who don't get enough sleep are more likely to have problems with attention, emotional control, and peer relationship.

Another study showed significant differences in 7-year-old children regarding executive function (including attention, working memory, reasoning, and problem-solving) depending on how much sleep they regularly received at younger ages.

Elsie Taveras, a pediatrics professor at Harvard Medical School and chief of general pediatrics at Massachusetts General Hospital for Children, led the study. She said, "We found that children who get an insufficient amount of sleep in their preschool and early school-age years have a higher risk of poor neurobehavioral function at around age 7."[5]

So, are you convinced? Poor sleep is a problem. We'll discuss why it's an issue and how to repair the damage done so you can get back on track to obtaining full health.

CIRCADIAN RHYTHMS

Do you have moments where you feel more alert throughout the day and other times when the drowsiness hits? Have you noticed those moments of energy or sleepiness tend to be around the same time? That's your circadian rhythm (also known as your sleep/wake cycle) running in your brain, cycling between windows of energy and sleepiness.

Most adults experience energy dips in the middle of the night while asleep, then again between about 1:00 and 3:00 p.m. These patterns may be different depending on your sleeping habits, like if you go to sleep late every night or wake up in the early hours each day. If you're dealing with sleep deprivation, you'll notice these slumps more than if you were getting enough sleep.

---

[5]   https://news.harvard.edu/gazette/story/2017/03/study-flags-later-risks-for-sleep-deprived-kids

A portion of your brain called the hypothalamus controls your circadian rhythm, but outside factors such as light or darkness can also affect your sleep/wake cycles. Your circadian rhythm is most effective when your sleep habits are consistent. If you're going to sleep and waking at different times each day, your circadian rhythm gets off track. It's best to try to stay consistent in your sleep times, even on the weekends.

SLEEP AND THE BRAIN

Have you ever gone to bed feeling so upset about something, and then you feel calm about the same thing in the morning? Or do you deal with irrational worries when you awake at unusual hours of the night?

You may be surprised by the role that adequate sleep has on your brain function. It's been proven that good sleep can decrease mental fatigue, improve memory, and control metabolism. However, researchers have found that to maintain proper cognitive function, seven hours of sleep is necessary.

The brain is hard at work while we sleep. It eliminates toxic waste byproducts that have amassed throughout the day. It recharges and reorganizes itself during those hours of rest, returning to normal function by the time you awaken. Every phase in the sleep cycle is vital for restoring and rejuvenating the brain for optimal function, so when sleep is disrupted, it affects your behavior, judgment, and cognitive function.

SLEEP AND THE IMMUNE SYSTEM

Have you heard the phrase, "I'm sick and tired of being sick and tired?" It turns out that the two coincide. People who don't sleep well are more likely to get sick after being exposed to a virus, and it also affects how fast they recover from illness.

Your immune system releases sleep-promoting proteins called cytokines. You need more of those when you have inflammation, stress, or an infection, but lack of sleep can decrease the production of cytokines.

Cells and antibodies that fight infection decline when you're sleep-deprived. You're also more at risk for cardiovascular disease, diabetes, and obesity when you deal with long-term lack of sleep.

So, in a nutshell, your body really needs good sleep. It's not enough to get more sleep—it needs to be quality sleep to provide you with the best benefits.[6]

SLEEP AND WEIGHT LOSS

There probably isn't a week that goes by when we don't have at least one new patient consultation where one of the patient's top three complaints is that they can't seem to lose weight. The typical conversation highlights that they have tried numerous diets, and they are beating themselves to death at the gym. They're left feeling frustrated because the approach that used to work doesn't anymore.

These same people are often tired and sluggish throughout the day and deal with a lot of stress. Almost everyone initially starts their weight-loss journey by reducing their calorie intake and working out for 1 hour or more 3-5 days a week. Most of these patients are convinced that their next move is to reduce calories even more and hit the gym one more day.

They are always surprised to hear that it may be time to go in a totally different direction. You can imagine the looks we get after telling patients they may be working out too much already.

---

[6]   https://www.mayoclinic.org/diseases-conditions/insomnia/expert-answers/lack-of-sleep/faq-20057757

A COMPLEX, INTERCONNECTED SYSTEM

Our body's metabolism is a complex and interconnected system, and this system craves balance. It requires careful attention to all aspects of the Simple 7 Lifestyle to function well and remain in a state of ease and health. Too little food is as dangerous as too much. Too much exercise can be as detrimental as not enough. So, what happens when a person is already working out too much and causing stress on their body, and then they decide to wake up an hour earlier or stay up an hour later to squeeze in that workout? Well, it can spell a metabolic "perfect storm."

Just how important is sleep? In an article published in JAMA, Bridget Kuehn provides an excellent summary of the importance of sleep and circadian rhythms in regulating our metabolic engines. Certain areas of the brain respond to natural (and artificial) light/dark cycles. When these areas of the brain are out of sync, it can alter our ability to regulate blood sugar, lead to obesity and diabetes, and lower our resting metabolic rate. These issues are compounded by the modern challenges of light pollution and the increasing use of electronic devices that emit the same wavelengths as the sun. These artificial lights can trigger disruptions of this internal body clock.

According to Eve Van Cauter, Ph.D., professor of medicine at the University of Chicago, our "sleep, circadian rhythms, and metabolism make up an inseparable triad." She says, "The work so far suggests that being sleep deprived and losing weight are contradictory. To optimize weight loss, you need to sleep."

So, if you are trying to lose a few pounds, remember that there's more to weight loss than just diet and exercise. Even though we live in a society where sleep is not very highly respected, it is critical to hormonal health and weight management.

HOW TO GET BETTER SLEEP

Now you know how vital good sleep is, but getting quality sleep is easier said than done, right?

If you're one of the many unlucky individuals who deal with sleep deprivation, there are so many things you can do to improve your sleep. We've provided a list of helpful tips that can vastly improve your sleep if you start implementing them now. Determine which suggestions will be easiest for you to begin with and start there.

TOP 10 TIPS TO IMPROVE YOUR SLEEP

1. **Sleep in complete darkness**. If there is too much electric light in your room, it can disrupt your circadian rhythm and your pineal gland's melatonin and serotonin production. If you must get up in the middle of the night for any reason, try to use as little light as possible or find a small night light with an amber or red bulb.

2. **Keep the temperature in the bedroom no higher than 70 degrees F**. Many people keep their homes and particularly the upstairs bedrooms too hot. This can disrupt the body's circadian rhythms and REM sleep cycles, impacting the quality of rest you feel the next morning.

3. **Reserve your bed for sleeping and connection.** If you are watching TV or doing work in bed, you may find it harder to relax and think of the bed as a place to sleep. It's best to move the TV completely out of the bedroom.

4. **Get to bed before 11pm.** Our body does a lot of recharging and recovering during the hours of 11 p.m. and 1 a.m. Your gallbladder also dumps toxins during this same period. If you're awake, the toxins back up into the liver, which then secondarily back up into your entire system and cause

further disruption of your health. Before the widespread use of electricity, people would go to bed shortly after sundown, as most animals do, and which nature intended for humans.

5. **Establish a bedtime routine.** This could include meditation, deep breathing, aromatherapy or essential oils, or indulging in a massage from your partner. It could include a hot shower or bath, journaling or reading something inspiring and motivational. The key is to find something that makes you feel relaxed, then repeat it each night to help release the day's tensions.

6. **Avoid light-emitting screens 2 hours before bed.** Put your work away and unplug from the stresses of life. This will give your mind a chance to unwind so you can go to sleep feeling calm rather than anxious about tomorrow's deadlines.

7. **Exercise in the morning.** Exercising for at least 30 minutes every day can help you fall asleep. However, don't exercise too close to bedtime, or it may keep you awake. Studies show exercising in the morning is the best if you can fit it in.

8. **Keep your sleep and wake times consistent.** Waking up and going to sleep at nearly the same time each night and day, even on weekends, will help to establish a rhythm in your hormones and brain chemistry.

9. **Avoid before-bed snacks, particularly grains and sugars.** This will raise blood sugar and inhibit sleep. Later, when blood sugar drops too low (hypoglycemia), you might wake up and not be able to fall back asleep. If you need to eat something, have a small serving of protein, fat, and a small amount of fruit.

10. **Listen to white noise or relaxation CDs.** Some people find white noise or nature sounds, such as the ocean or forest, to be soothing for sleep.

TAKE ACTION: IDEAL BEDTIME ROUTINE

You know of all the benefits from obtaining more sleep. Now it's time to make your own game plan! See the list from above and choose three or four tips you could personally work on.

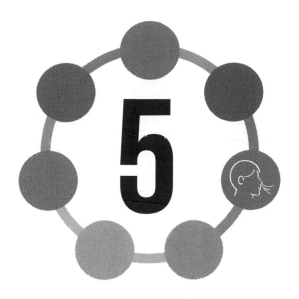

BREATHE WELL

Breath is the most fundamental element of life. We can survive days without food or water, but we can't last more than a few minutes without breathing.

Could there be anything more obvious than the essential nature of breathing? Many people might say it is so obvious that it wouldn't be necessary to include it in a list of healthy habits. The current prevailing medical thought is that there isn't much to discuss around this topic. It doesn't matter if it is ten times a minute, twenty times through your mouth, or through your nose or a mechanical ventilator; as long as a person can breathe enough oxygen to stay alive, that is all that is needed.

But just because we breathe thousands of times per day doesn't mean that we are doing it correctly. Millions of people suffer from a wide range of health conditions brought about by faulty breathing habits.

We could say that simply eating enough calories can keep a person alive but focusing on food quality can lead to longevity and vitality. The same goes for breath. Moving around during our daily activities is better than doing nothing, but much more beneficial to move correctly and exercise efficiently. The same could be said for sleep, play, relationships, and our mental and emotional frames. Similar to these other habits, it turns out that there are secrets of health potential buried under the surface if we are willing to look.

By incorporating some of the breathwork exercises we'll share in this book, millions of people have improved their chronic diseases to renewed health.

AN ANCIENT ART

The study of breathing isn't anything new. Ancient civilizations have known the importance of breathing correctly, and many of them have left records of how breath was used as a part of their healing arts.

4,000-year-old Chinese Taoist texts taught that "Breath must be taken in through the nose. Never do otherwise, for breath would be in danger and illness would set in."

Native Americans believed that breath inhaled through the mouth sapped the body of strength, deformed the face, and caused stress and disease, while breathing through the nose kept the body strong, made a face beautiful, and prevented disease.

Although ancient health texts worldwide give ample attention to the profound impact that the quality of our breathing impacts our health, western science is only now starting to prove many of these ancient practices.

Since our goal in this book is to capitalize on simple, simple behaviors that are available to everyone with little to no cost, we'll teach you some straightforward yet practical breathing techniques you can easily incorporate into your life. But to help you fully understand the impact of these exercises, we'll first discuss the basics of breathing.

WHAT DOES BREATHING DO?

At its most basic scientific explanation, breathing is simply about an exchange of gasses. Our cells need a constant supply of oxygen to fire our cellular furnace, and in that process, one of the byproducts is carbon dioxide. Our red blood cells are the transportation vehicles for these gasses. The only way to unload an oxygen molecule from the red blood cell is to switch it with a molecule of carbon dioxide.

This transportation of billions of molecules in and out of our bodies also profoundly influences every organ and system of our body, telling them when to work and when to rest. The presence of these molecules affects our heart rate, digestion, brain activity, mood, and much more.

Our breathing also has a mechanical and structural benefit to our health. Our breath is driven by the contraction and downward tug of the diaphragm, one of the body's largest muscles. This essential muscle runs across our thorax and serves to separate our chest cavity from our abdominal cavity. When it contracts, it pushes downward and creates a larger volume of space in our chest cavity. The diaphragm's movement creates a vacuum effect and draws in air to fill the lungs and occupy the area that has been created. When the diaphragm relaxes, it returns to its original position, which expels the carbon dioxide out of the lungs.

As our diaphragm repeatedly moves up and down like a large piston, that movement squeezes the largest vessels of our lymphatic system. This squeezing action works as a pump to move toxins and cellular wastes from the lymph system into the liver to be detoxified.

So, our lungs are vital organs of detoxification, first through the removal of carbon dioxide and secondly through the action on the lymphatic system.

BROKEN BREATHING?

Before we explain why learning to breathe better is worthy of your conscious effort and time, we need to explain the negative health impacts of improper breathing and why we have become a nation of poor breathers in the first place.

Anthropological research shows that over the past 10,000 years or so, the shape of our skulls has dramatically changed. There are several theories as to the reasons behind these changes, the most likely among them being that we've made significant changes in our diets with the advent of agriculture. Researchers that studied native populations that were relatively untouched by modern diets and lifestyles noticed that these populations had wide mouths, with plenty of room for beautifully straight teeth, strong jawbone structures, and large, open sinus passages. When these people switched to modern diets, their faces began to change within only a few generations.

The average modern human's skull is now much narrower than our ancient ancestors. Many people in our society have mouths so small that their teeth are crowded and uneven without enough room for their "wisdom teeth" to fit. The roof of our mouths, called the palate, has gone from flat and wide to highly arched and narrow. This high palate encroaches into the sinus space, decreasing the physical size and increasing the likelihood of blockages.

THE MODERN MOUTHBREATHER

All these physical changes make it difficult to breathe properly through our noses. Allergies and other conditions that congest the sinuses make it so we're much more likely to breathe through our mouths rather than our noses.

And that is where one of the major problems lies. It turns out there is a surprising difference between the air we breathe through our nose and that which we breathe through our mouths.

When we breathe through our noses, the air is warmed, humidified, pressurized, and filtered. Breathing through our mouths can cause dental issues like periodontal disease, bad breath, and even cavities.

Obstructed sinuses and mouth breathing have also been strongly implicated in snoring and sleep apnea, affecting more and more adults and even young children.

Another challenge we face is that we typically breathe at a faster rate under stress. This evolutionary response is associated with our fight or flight response. Our nervous system perceives that we're in danger and quickly adapts our body to run. It only makes sense that part of that response would be to increase our heart rate and breathing rate to get more energy to our muscles. But when the perceived threats are chronic, these chemical and physical changes don't serve us well. We end up breathing faster and less deeply, leading to inefficient breaths.

Author Patrick McKeown calls this "overbreathing." In his book, *The Oxygen Advantage*, he has the following simple self-assessment quiz:

- Do you sometimes breathe through your mouth as you go about your daily activities?
- Do you breathe through your mouth during sleep? (If you're not sure, do you wake up with a dry mouth?)
- Do you snore or hold your breath during sleep?
- Can you visibly notice your breathing during rest? To find out, look at your breathing right now. Spend a minute observing the movement of your chest or abdomen as you take each breath. The more movement you see, the heavier your breath.
- When you observe your breathing, do you see more movements from the chest than from the abdomen?
- Do you regularly sigh throughout the day? (While one sigh every now and again is not an issue, regular sighing is enough to maintain chronic overbreathing.)
- Do you sometimes hear your breathing during rest?
- Do you experience symptoms resulting from habitual overbreathing, such as nasal congestion, tightening of the airways, fatigue, dizziness, or light-headedness?

Learning to slow our breathing and bring awareness to deep breathing is often the fastest way to lower our stress and anxiety levels. Proper breathing habits can improve athletic performance, improve metabolism and weight loss, and increase nitrous oxide, enhancing circulation by over 600%.

BREATHING BASICS

The most foundational principle of proper breathing is to inhale through the nose as much as possible. Next, it's best to focus on techniques that slow down our breathing and encourage deeper breaths that engage the diaphragm and expand the abdomen.

According to ancient practices and modern science, the optimal breathing rate is a 6-second inhalation and a 6-second exhalation. Any time you find yourself feeling stressed, it can be helpful to bring awareness to your breathing for a minute or two.

Count slowly to six as you inhale and exhale. We've noticed that even though we aren't perfect all of the time, focusing on this pattern at key times during the day can have a dramatic effect and create a new habit.

TYPES OF BREATHING EXERCISES

A variety of breathing exercises or practices have been developed over the centuries. Here are a few of the most accessible and simple techniques to help contribute to a healthy lifestyle.

DIAPHRAGMATIC BREATHING

Diaphragmatic breathing expands the abdomen and contracts the diaphragm (a muscle found at the base of the lungs), leading to deep, refreshing breaths. This type of breathing is a general practice for meditation and relaxation.

ALTERNATE NOSTRIL BREATHING

Alternate nostril breathing involves alternating between breathing and exhaling through each nostril with the support of the thumb and ring fingers to close each nostril one at a time. This technique can help balance the brain and nerve system and reduce the "fight or flight" response.

SLOW-PACED BREATHING (6X6, 2X4X6, 4X4X4)

This technique involves intentionally slowing the breathing rate, often with the help of an audio recording or breathing app. The intention is to have approximately 6-second inhalation and 6-second exhalation.

The 2x4x6 breathing technique is a variation of the slow-paced breathing technique and is a great way to calm anxiety. Start by inhaling for two seconds, holding the breath for four seconds, and then exhaling to the count of six. One more approach is to inhale to the count of four, hold for four more seconds, and then exhale for four seconds and hold for 4 seconds. This is often called "box breathing."

TUMMO OR "WIM HOF" BREATHING

Tummo breathing is an ancient practice repopularized by the "iceman" Wim Hof, an amazing Dutchman who has set out to prove the power of breathwork to enable him to accomplish amazing feats of human endurance and exposure. He has a specific approach to breathwork wherein you do deep 1-second inhalation and 1-second exhalation for a total of 30-seconds. This is followed by 30-90 seconds of breath-hold on exhalation, followed immediately by 15-seconds of breath-hold on inhalation. This entire sequence is then repeated two more times. Learn more at wimhofmethod.com.

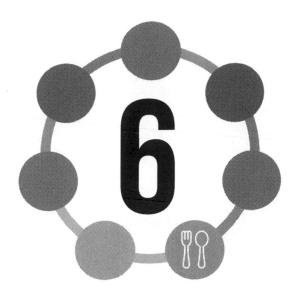

EAT WELL

TAMMIE'S GROCERY STORE EXPERIENCE

On my way home from work late one night, I remembered that the cupboards were bare, and the refrigerator was empty. If I didn't stop at the grocery store before returning home, my family members would wake up with hungry tummies, and there wouldn't be anything to nourish them.

As I began the methodical trek down the aisles, I heard an emotionally distressed child screaming in the distance. Immediately I thought, "Oh, that poor mom."

The child continued to cry and scream, and her distress echoed throughout the store the entire time I was shopping. Eventually I came face to face with a very flustered mom and sobbing child. I was shocked to see the following scene: this exhausted mom dragged her upset child by the arm behind her while also pushing an overflowing cart.

Finally, I finished my shopping and headed for the checkout line. It was late enough now that only one lane was open. As I approached the line, I heard the now-familiar wail of the worn-out child. I took my place in line and noticed that the toddler was now on the floor performing an elaborate tantrum while her mom searched through a giant binder of coupons to save some extra pennies.

I noticed the items in the shopping cart—packages, bottles, boxes, and cans of non-nourishing foods. When I heard "buy one, get one free," "save 55 cents," "Free with purchase," I made a powerful connection to the child on the floor and the items in the cart.

Without a doubt, I believe, just as eighteenth-century French physician Julien Offray De Lamettrie stated, "The human body is a machine that winds up its own springs…Without proper food, the soul languishes, raves, and dies with faintness."

As I looked at the cart again, I realized it had no signs of life. Nothing in that cart was living; therefore, there was nothing for the little body on the floor to wind up its springs. I concluded that there could be a connection between the distress I had heard since I entered the store that night and the lack of nourishment in that cart. The child could not voice it and did not realize it, but her subconscious knew it.

The cart was loaded to the point of overflowing, so full that the little girl couldn't even sit in it. I felt that she knew deep down in her little body that she was hungry, and the things in that cart were not going to satisfy that hunger. She was going home with food that would not nourish or sustain her body machine.

This "raving" and "languishing" took place there on the grocery store floor, all at the price of saving $60 in coupons. What a price to pay for savings! What if, instead, the mother did as Lamettrie suggests: "Give but good nourishment to the body, pour into its tubes vigorous juices, then the soul generous of these, arms itself with courage. What a vast power there is in repast… But as we are cheerful, or brave; all depends on the manner of winding up our machine."

This trip to the grocery store was the springboard for my desire to share what I know with others. This is why I do what I do, why

I share recipes and meal plans, why I teach classes and coach. It is why I help people understand that you can eat healthy foods and stick to your budget.

Cooking from scratch is not difficult; it is only a change in mindset. I can purchase the raw ingredients to create a meal that can also be found premade in the grocery store's freezer section, in a cardboard box, or aluminum can.

The difference is the raw ingredients are whole and living foods that have the essential building blocks to nurture and grow my body and my children's bodies. The frozen and canned foods too often contain ingredients and preservatives that don't nourish bodies.

This mom hadn't done anything to harm her child purposefully. She likely didn't know there was a better way. Many children grow up in our country with full bellies but without the essential nutrients their bodies and brains need to grow and thrive.

THE ULTIMATE GOAL: JUST. EAT. REAL. FOOD.

This mother that Tammie observed in the store certainly wasn't alone in feeling unsure of the best nutrition practices. We've found that 90% of our patients are confused about nutrition. It makes sense with all the contention and conflicting advice among the different camps. How can you know what's right?

Our goal with this chapter is to clear up the confusion and help you feel confident in the decisions you make concerning your nutrition.

ROLE OF DIET AND NUTRITION

Nutrition is one of the primary pillars of optimal health and wellness. One could make the case that general health starts here. The quality, quantity, and frequency of eating has more impact on your overall health than anything else.

An estimated 95% of all illness is related to cumulative negative stresses we experience. It's no secret that "stress" changes the way we eat. People dealing with stress tend to eat foods high in sweets and starches that quickly convert to sugar in the in the bloodstream. This quick fuel can keep us going in emergencies but too frequently becomes our fuel of choice for non-emergencies. If you have chronic health concerns, addressing your diet is a critical component of healing.

When we are under stress, predictable physiological changes occur in which the mechanisms that control blood sugar levels are taxed.

THE DANGERS OF PROCESSED FOODS & DRINKS

So, what's the big deal with processed foods, the kinds that over-loaded the stressed-out mom's cart in the grocery store? Everyone eats them, right?

The problem with a lot of the food found in boxes, bags, and cans is that it contains what we call "Frankenfoods," or any genet-ically modified food made in a lab or factory. Frankenfoods are packed with unhealthy preservatives, trans fats, chemicals, sodium, and other artificial ingredients. Sometimes they're even packaged in a way that makes you believe they're healthy or natural, but they're not.

The best diet consists mostly of food that could be picked, hunted, or gathered for optimal health. It may not always feel simple to determine what foods are acceptable and which you should avoid, so we'll dive into the harmful foods that we highly recommend you completely eliminate.

ARTIFICIAL COLORS AND SWEETENERS

Too many packaged foods contain harmful artificial ingredients. Avoid synthetic dyes like FD&C Red No. 40, Tartrazine, or Blue No. 1. Exclude artificial sweeteners like saccharin, aspartame, or sucralose from your diet.

7Artificial ingredients haven't been around all that long. In a sense, the food industry has turned our society into guinea pigs to see how our bodies react to these artificial coloring and sweeteners. And in truth, our bodies don't respond well to them.

Look for dyes from natural sources (like paprika, saffron, or annatto) or forget the coloring altogether. When it comes to sweeteners, pick those that come from natural sources (like honey, maple syrup, and even sugar) over the artificial stuff, but always consume them in moderation.

REFINED SWEETENERS

Refined sweeteners aren't all that bad; it's the quantity consumed that has become a big problem. Sugar is no longer reserved for special occasions anymore and instead is lurking in almost everything you purchase. Instead of being labeled simply as "sugar," you'll find many variants in packaged foods, including corn syrup, high-fructose corn syrup, cane juice, brown rice syrup, or whatever creative word or initials are on the label.

Rely on natural sweeteners like honey and maple syrup since they are mostly "processed" in nature and contain some trace nutrients. However, it's important to remember that "sugar is sugar," no matter what you choose. Even if you go the more natural route (which we highly recommend), that by no means gives you the green light to turn up the bottle. It's also helpful to buy foods "plain," like yogurt, for example, and sparingly sweeten them yourself to make sure things don't get out of hand.

FACTORY FARMED MEAT AND SEAFOOD

Factory farms raise animals in overcrowded and confined quarters and feed the animals unnatural diets. According to author Michael Pollan, "You are what you eat eats too." This means that the diet of the animals we eat has a bearing on the nutritional quality and healthfulness of the food itself, whether meat, milk, or eggs. Some of our food animals, such as cows and sheep, are ruminants that evolved to eat grass; if they eat too many seeds, they become sick. Grain-fed cattle often require a lot of antibiotics. Even animals that do well on grain, such as chickens and pigs, are much healthier when they have access to green plants.

When an animal is healthy, their meat and eggs are too. For most of our food animals, a diet of grass means much healthier fats (more omega-3s and fewer omega-6s and saturated fat) in their meat, milk, and eggs, as well as appreciably higher levels of vitamins and antioxidants.

Factory farms also hurt the environment and raise animals in an inhumane manner. Shop your local farmer's market for humanely raised and pastured animal products. We highly recommend searching for free-range/grass-finished ranchers to supply your beef and purchase wild-caught fish. If you are concerned about the higher cost, try eating less meat. Many recipes still taste the same with half the meat they call for.

INGREDIENTS YOU WOULDN'T USE AT HOME

Rather than memorizing a detailed list of chemicals to avoid in packaged foods, we'll make this one easy for you: don't buy food made with ingredients you wouldn't cook with at home. The ingredients you want to avoid are usually easy to spot on ingredient labels; they're words you wouldn't be able to spell or maybe even pronounce.

Stick with simple products made from a short list of real food ingredients. Better yet, make your foods from scratch. You can save money when you start making your own sauces, seasoning, and salad dressings.

REFINED OILS

While olive oil and other cold-pressed oils have been around for centuries, refined alternatives like shortening, soybean oil, seed oils, and vegetable oils (canola, safflower, sunflower, corn oil) are relatively new on the market. The food industry produces these oils as a cheap alternative to high-quality oils. These highly processed vegetable oils are heated at high temperatures, causing them to become damaged and rancid. They are then "cleaned" up with chemicals and hydrogenated to improve their flavor and shelf stability.

Fats are good for us, but we need to consume fats we're naturally intended to, like butter, ghee, olive oil, unrefined coconut oil, avocado oil, and even pastured lard. These fats can also be damaged if not processed correctly, so look for words like "cold-pressed," "organic," "virgin," or "unrefined" on the label.

IMITATION FOODS

Imitation foods are those that pretend to be something they're not, like margarine, processed cheese products, imitation crab meat, pancake syrup, and lemonade powder. The bottom line is that imitation foods are a highly processed fake version of the real thing. Buy the true versions of foods like real butter, cheese, crab, pure maple syrup, and make lemonade with real lemons (not artificial powder).

Real food is self-contained in a form that works harmoniously to deliver vitamins and minerals to the body. Processed food doesn't work that way; it's just ingredients put together to create a desired product. The ingredients may not even offer any nutrients to the body. Again, if you could hunt it, pick it, milk it, gather it, or fish it, you should be able to eat it.

OUR CURRENT DIET DILEMMA

Science has conclusively proven that virtually every chronic disease known to man is rooted in diet and that we have the power to change how we live and function if we take control of our lifestyle. We don't have to be a nation of tired, overweight, stressed out, and depressed people!

Have you heard, "You are what you eat"? Why is that precious gem of truth so hard to remember when it comes to healing our bodies?

We've discussed why you should avoid processed foods, so now we'll give you the "skinny" on the foods that should form the basis of your diet for the rest of your life.

Our entire society is deceived by all sorts of corporate marketers, fad diets, and quick fixes. It's no longer clear what is the best food for us to eat and what will provide the most nourishment to our bodies.

We know other roadblocks and challenges can thwart our progress on the journey to a better diet, including the following:

- **Time crunches** – We've become a fast-paced society, dependent on fast food and quick calories.
- **We've lost the art of cooking** – Many people have never learned to prepare meals from scratch. Even the traditional "Sunday dinner" comes from boxes and bags these days.
- **Instant gratification** – We have difficulty with processes that take time to yield results. While many people do see quick results from dietary change, the benefits are measured over months, years, and decades.
- **No system and no support** – We often embark on dietary change without a support network or a clear plan to follow. We hodge-podge various ideas together, don't tell anyone, try to do it on our own, and then fail miserably.
- **Bad habits** – Maybe you grew up eating a certain way and even though you know it's not the most nutritious for your body, you have a hard time letting go of bad eating habits.

BECKY'S STORY

When Becky came to work with us, she was significantly overweight, fatigued, and burned out. She was also suffering from chronic migraine headaches and a troubling autoimmune disease. She had patches of dry, irritated skin all over her body, and she could barely concentrate on her work. To add insult to the situation, her children were following in her footsteps. She could see she was headed in the wrong direction in a *big* way. She wanted to change, but fear and confusion paralyzed her.

It's always a bit daunting to sit with someone like Becky, someone who needs a comprehensive overhaul of her entire approach to health. Thank goodness she had the one essential ingredient – commitment. She was wholly committed to her health and to creating a different life for her and her family.

Western medicine has failed people like Becky. They don't have a little pill or procedure that can solve these multifactorial conditions. The answer for Becky, and by extension millions just like her, was to take charge of her life through her diet!

Becky was instructed in the Simple 7 Lifestyle principles, and she embraced them with childlike confidence and trust that things would work for her. And they did work!

Within a matter of days, she had begun to shed dramatic amounts of weight. Initially, most of her weight loss was water weight due to fluid retention secondary to eating foods she was highly allergic to.

Soon, however, the fat started melting off. Within four months, Becky had already shed the burden of over 40 lbs. Her migraines had virtually disappeared, her energy was sky high, her skin cleared up, and the people in her life noticed her dramatic transformation.

DON'T FORGET WATER

Changing your diet will make massive improvements to your health but increasing your water intake needs to be part of that change.

So many people struggle to drink enough water each day, but if they knew the dangers of dehydration, chances are they'd make more of an effort to drink more.

Your body uses water regularly to carry out its normal functions. When you don't have enough water to replenish what your body uses, you get dehydrated.

Dehydration can occur when we simply don't drink enough. It worsens in people who have severe diarrhea or vomiting, don't drink enough water in hot weather, or take medication that increases dehydration.

There may be long periods when you think you don't need water because you don't feel thirsty, but often, we don't feel the urge to drink until we're already dehydrated.

STAY HYDRATED, STAY HEALTHY

Hydration is essential for optimal health. We can go about a month without food, but we would only live two or three days without water. Our bodies are made of about 60% water, and every cell, tissue, and organ needs water to function. Staying hydrated can prevent the problems of dehydration, but there are several more ways water benefits the body:

- Transports nutrients and oxygen to cells
- Keeps your skin elasticity healthy
- Regulates your body temperature
- Helps you properly digest food and eliminate waste regularly
- Lubricates your joints
- Eliminates toxins
- Protects organs and keeps them functioning properly
- Energizes your muscles
- Enables you to think more clearly
- Combats hunger and makes you feel full
- Aids in weight loss

HOW MUCH SHOULD WE DRINK?

Drink water throughout the day and avoid feeling thirsty. You should drink about a quart of water for every 50 pounds you weigh. If this seems daunting, start your day with a big drink of water and slowly work your way up to consuming more throughout the day. If plain water just doesn't hit the spot for you, try infusing your water with fruit, veggies, and fresh herbs.

Being thirsty can make you feel tired, weak, unable to focus, and lead to headaches. Our brain may even send a signal that feels like "I'm hungry," but it really means, "I'm super thirsty!" Try drinking a big glass of water before grabbing a snack or eat a snack with high water content, like cucumbers, watermelon, celery, apples, citrus, and leafy greens. Avoid all foods and drinks that take water from the body. Dehydrating foods include soda, fried foods, and sugar.

Sometimes we just don't think to drink water, but it's essential to get enough each day. Here are a few tips to help you remember to drink more:

- Every time you get a text or email notification, take a drink of water.
- Fill up a reusable water bottle and keep it with you all the time.
- Put a rubber band around the center of your water bottle, one for every full bottle that you need to drink that day. Each time you finish a bottle, move the rubber band to the top or put it around your wrist. Keep drinking until all the rubber bands have moved.

5 REASONS TO DRINK WATER IN THE MORNING

Imagine not drinking any liquid for the next eight hours. That's exactly what we do while we sleep. Our bodies don't make or store water, so we slowly get dehydrated when we don't drink for an extended period. This is why it's essential to re-hydrate your body as soon as you wake up in the morning.

The following are the top five reasons to hydrate first thing in the morning.

1. **Combat dehydration.** You just went 7-8 hours without drinking any water! Your body may not be giving you the signals that it's thirsty, but it probably is. Drink at least 16 ounces of water upon waking up. Better yet, shoot for 32 ounces!

2. **Fire up your metabolism.** A study published by the *Journal of Clinical Endocrinology and Metabolism* found that drinking at least 16 ounces of water increased the metabolic rate in healthy men and women by 30 percent. This boost occurred within 10 minutes of drinking and lasted about 40 minutes. This research could also imply that our metabolism will remain active if we continue drinking throughout the day.

3. **Flush out toxins.** Your liver and kidneys do a fantastic job of cleansing and ridding your body of toxins if your intake of fluids is adequate. Your skin will also get rid of toxins if there is enough fluid for it to sweat. Getting fluids into your body right after waking up will help your body flush out toxins first thing in the morning.

4. **Fuel your brain.** Your brain is made up of 75 percent water. When you're not adequately hydrated, your brain operates on less fuel, and you can feel drained, experience fatigue, mood fluctuations, or headaches.

5. **You'll eat less.** The signal that we get for thirst and hunger is the same. When most people get that signal, they eat. Instead of eating, take a big drink of water and wait a little while to see if your hunger pangs return or if you were just thirsty.

THE 7 FOOD RULES FOR HEALTH

1-DRINK ENOUGH WATER

When people think of nutrients, it is rare that they even think of the essential nutrient we need, good old water. Our bodies are 60% water, and our brains are closer to 75%. Every single cell requires a medium of water to transport every other nutrient around our body.

2-EAT WHOLE, REAL FOOD WHENEVER POSSIBLE

We know that there are times when "good" food is scarce (like at the neighborhood party or on long road trips). The best thing to do in these situations is to plan ahead. Offer to bring something to the neighborhood party and pack your own food for long road trips. If that's not possible, always choose foods with the least amount of processing. We like to ask if the food we are eating could have conceivably been hunted, fished, picked, or harvested.

3-EAT RIGHT FOR YOUR METABOLISM

You are the best scientist when it comes to how your body reacts to foods. Pay attention to your energy and your overall sense of wellbeing after you eat, and you will come to understand how much protein, carbs, and fats you need for optimal energy during the day.

4-DON'T SKIP MEALS

There is something to be said for periodic, intermittent fasting, but for the most part, we need to eat on a regular enough basis to maintain blood sugar and energy requirements.

5-EAT AT REGULAR INTERVALS

For most people, we find that three balanced meals work just right. Some do better when they fast through breakfast and eat two meals per day with an occasional snack if necessary. Experiment with what works better for you.

6-AVOID ALL ALLERGENS AND SENSITIVITIES

It is crucial to eliminate 100% of the foods that you are reacting to. If you give your body time and the proper environment to heal, it is possible to eliminate food sensitivities. This requires sufficient time and a careful reintroduction process, especially if you are making a conscious effort to heal and repair the gut.

7-FOR ALL OTHER FOODS, FOLLOW THE 90:10 RULE

By following a whole-food diet 90% of the time, we are going to have good long-term success and create a great relationship with food. It's okay to let your guard down on special occasions if they are only 10% of the time rather than a daily occurrence.

Make sure you are eating a diverse diet. Do your best not to get stuck in a rut of eating the same foods day after day. Diversity keeps your gut and your brain happy.

SET YOURSELF UP FOR SUCCESS

Take small manageable steps rather than one big drastic change. Approach these small steps with commitment, decide why you want to make these changes. Say to yourself, "If I make these changes, then I can _____." We are more committed and motivated to change if there is a purpose.

- **Simplify** - Focus on finding foods you love and easy recipes that incorporate fresh real food ingredients. Gradually, your diet will become healthier and more delicious.
- **Start Slow** - Make changes to your eating habits over time. Trying to make your diet healthy overnight isn't realistic. Changing everything at once usually leads to feelings of overwhelm or giving up on your new eating plan.
- **Involve Others** - Include all the members of your family, even extended family. When people know you're making changes and why you're doing it they will be more likely to accept the changes and usually do their best to offer support.
- **Every Change Matters** - Any change you make toward improvement matters. You don't have to be perfect right now! Don't let your missteps derail you. Remind yourself that every healthy food choice is building health not tearing it down.
- **Clean Out Your Kitchen** – Remove things that tempt you and won't nourish you. It's much easier to eat nutritiously when you're surrounded by good foods and when less than stellar foods are out of your home.

TAKE ACTION: 7 DAYS TO CHANGE YOUR LIFE

In seven days, you could truly change your life in a way that would bring more vitality. Follow the daily plan below, focusing on the challenge for each day, and in a week, you'll see how easy this change can be!

DAY 1: REAL HYDRATION

Today's simple focus will be to drink more water. Water makes up about 60% of your body. Your cells, tissues, and organs need water to function properly. You need water to digest, cleanse, and eliminate. Our bodies also need to rehydrate after sweating, crying, breathing, and producing saliva. Remember to aim for a quart of water to every

50 lbs. of body weight. Try eating water-dense foods like cucumbers, watermelon, celery, apples, Romaine lettuce, and citrus.

DAY 2: VEGGIES AND FRUIT

Eat veggies and fruit, especially in that order. We should have 9-11 servings every day. Try eating two servings with every meal this week. Feel free to eat veggies in unlimited amounts during the day, but it's best to limit yourself to 2-3 servings of fruit per day. Too much sugar, even natural fruit sugar, can be too much for your body to handle. Veggies and fruits give us vitamins, minerals, fiber, and disease-fighting phytonutrients.

DAY 3: TRY SOMETHING NEW

Find a new whole real food that you've never tried before and give it a try! A fun place to try new foods is at the farmer's market because there are always samples. Try at least one new recipe each week. Involve the family in food preparation. If they make it, they will usually want to taste it too!

DAY 4: EAT REAL FAT

Replace the hydrogenated, trans-fat filled refined oils that might be in your pantry with real healthy fats. Use coconut oil for baking and cooking anything over medium heat. Use olive oil for salad dressings and low heat cooking. Include raw nuts and seeds in your diet. Healthy fats are essential to nourish your brain, heart, and every cell in your body.

DAY 5: GET RID OF REFINED SWEETENERS

It's not what you eat some of the time but what you eat *most* of the time that makes a difference. We all like a sweet treat from time to time, but the average American consumes an average of 140 pounds of sugar per year. Why would anyone eat that much sugar? Well, maybe they don't realize they're eating that much. Refined sweeteners are addictive and deplete our body of vital minerals and enzymes. The good news is when you feed your body whole real food, it will stop craving refined sweeteners.

Look in your pantry and your fridge. Get rid of the foods that contain refined sweeteners and replace them with healthier alternatives.

DAY 6: PROPER PORTIONS

Did you know your entire meal should be only 2-4 handfuls of food? Use smaller plates and bowls to help you eat smaller portions. Don't eat until you feel full or stuffed. Take your time, wait, and listen for your body to send you signals. Save any leftovers to make preparing lunch for the next day easy!

DAY 7: FIVE INGREDIENTS OR LESS

When you are purchasing food from the store, try to find items that contain no more than five ingredients that you can pronounce. Foods made from scratch in your own kitchen may have more than five ingredients, but you know what those are and probably where they came from.

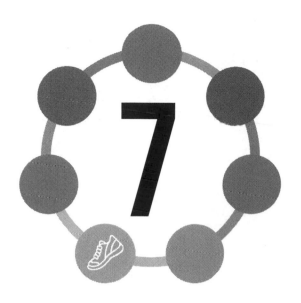

MOVE WELL

MOVE IT OR LOSE IT

Think about a time when you felt physically ill. Maybe you were sick with food poisoning, you had a terrible migraine, or you were in bed with the flu. When you were going through these moments, there was probably a lot you would've done to get better as quickly as possible. Or if there had been something you could have done to prevent yourself from getting sick, you probably would've taken that opportunity in a heartbeat.

Now think about the future. What if there were things you could do now that could prevent you from dealing with excruciating pain later? We're guessing your future self would give a heartfelt thank you to the past version of yourself for taking care to avoid the pain.

You already know there are things you can do to prevent future pain or disease, but sometimes it's hard to think about how our current actions (or inactions) will affect us in the future.

Exercise is one of those things we may struggle to take part in, but we know it will benefit us in the future. But *how much* can it help our bodies?

Regular exercise has consistently been shown in peer-reviewed studies to lower your risk of heart disease and increase the chances of survival after a heart attack. Researchers from Johns Hopkins in Baltimore and Henry Ford in Detroit reviewed data on over 2000 adults who had undergone previous stress tests and later had heart attacks. Their results found that those who were less physically fit before their first heart attack had an increased risk of dying within the first year following their heart attack. Increasing fitness levels after a heart attack also improves long-term health outcomes.

FOUNDATIONAL ACTIVITY

Our modern lifestyle is much more sedentary than societies in the past. We sit more and move our bodies less. Research proves that even those who exercise an hour every day can lose the benefits from that exercise if they remain sedentary for the rest of the day. Going for that jog or taking part in the spin class is great, but those activities don't do much good if you sit for the rest of the day.

We focus on the importance of whole-body movement, which is not quite the same as exercise and fitness because the end goal is slightly different. The goal with whole-body movement is to learn how to maintain health over a lifetime, not just to get fit, build muscle, or become an athlete.

First, we focus mainly on building lean muscle and maintaining pain-free, healthy movement throughout your life. This focus also helps to turn on your metabolism so that you can maintain a lean body.

While there are a variety of meanings to the phrase "move it or lose it", we assert that one meaning is that if we don't move our bodies, we lose lean muscle, and the amount of lean muscle we have is a powerful marker of overall longevity because lean muscle creates the metabolic engine that drives our hormones, energy balance and body composition.

You may have heard the phrase, "Sitting is the new smoking." What we're finding now is that being sedentary is just as damaging to our cardiovascular system and our whole-body health as smoking is. So, you might think you're doing great because you're not a smoker, but if you're sitting 9.5 hours like the average American is, it's causing the same damage and leading to the same degenerative diseases - like cancer and heart disease. It is one of the most significant risk factors for chronic disease and early death. When we don't move, we lose lean body mass and basically accelerate our demise.

Many people who want to lose weight attempt to exercise their way out of a problem, but that doesn't usually work. The foundation of all healthy movement is simply being active. How many steps we take, how many flights of stairs we walk up, how many times we go from sitting to standing to walking. These basic movements are vital.

Suppose we were to equate diet to activity and supplementation to exercise. In that case, basic movement is the equivalent of our daily food intake. Additional exercises we do, such as strength, endurance, and flexibility, are the equivalent of a supplement on top of that diet.

STRENGTH

To maintain a healthy body, we must build strength. We develop and maintain lean muscle by causing the body to break it down and rebuild it. We must demand our muscles to work to build strength.

ENDURANCE

Our bodies also need endurance, which is the capacity of our body to do an activity for a prolonged period. We often think of this simply as cardiovascular endurance, but muscular endurance is also critical. Many people like to do a strength workout one day and a cardio workout the next day; we'll talk about combining those exercises to build endurance.

FLEXIBILITY

When you go to the gym, you'll likely see plenty of people lifting weights or sweating on a treadmill or elliptical machine. How often do you see people stretching?

We often push flexibility to the backburner, but all our joints need to move through their full range of motion every day with ease and freedom.

Most of us gradually lose range of motion in our body without realizing it because we don't experience pain. We just can't move as much as we used to. We could touch our toes in the past, and now when we stretch, we reach our shins or maybe our knees. Some people may not be able to look up or turn their heads from side to side. These kinds of issues can be avoided or improved with daily or weekly flexibility movements.

7 PRIMAL MOVEMENTS

These facets of healthy movement all rely on seven primal movements which our bodies make all the time.

1. **Bending**
   Think of simple "hinge" types of movements like flexing at your hips to allow your arms to reach down to the floor. Bend your elbows and knees as well.

2. **Squating**
   Bend your knees or hips down toward the floor, keeping the back relatively straight. In Asia, it's not uncommon to see adults squatting down and resting in this position. Instead of sitting down on the ground, people in the Asian culture can often remain in a squatted position for hours. Squatting isn't a movement we make very often in Western culture, but it's an essential movement for us to regain.

3. **Lunging**

   Take a long stride forward and drop the back knee close to the ground, keeping your torso straight up. As you do the lunge, try rotating or twisting the core of the body from right to left.

4. **Rotating**

   Many people do rotational movements when they play a sport like tennis, racquetball, pickleball, baseball, or golf, but most people don't rotate both directions in those sports. Try to rotate the body both ways every day.

5. **Pushing**

   The classic exercise for pushing would be like a bench press, but a bench press is not a functional movement. We'll rarely have our back up against a fixed wall and try to push something. In real life, if we want to push something, we also have to stabilize our weight with our bodies. Imagine trying to free a car that is stuck in the snow. You have to generate all that energy with a stable core, and you have to stay fixed to the ground. Pushing, even if it's an upper-body activity, can be a whole-body movement.

6. **Pulling**

   In the past, humans climbed trees and developed upper muscle strength. This kind of activity decompresses the spine by the force of gravity. When we push down on the spine and hang by our arms, we can open up the spine. Pulling objects toward us can also do this; for example, try pulling down weight from a bar over your head.

7. **Walking**

   The seventh primal movement is walking. You can also incorporate jogging, running, or sprinting.

YOGA

Yoga is a powerful, multifaceted form of movement we'd highly recommend you try. You don't have to join a yoga studio or dive into Eastern religion. There are plenty of free videos on the internet to help guide you.

Yoga is an amazing system that's been developed for thousands of years; there's profound wisdom in this type of movement. At the purely physical level, yoga allows our bodies to move through full ranges of motion and develop core strength and stability. You can also do it as a meditation to help lower stress, anxiety, and inflammation. Yoga can also help improve flexibility and balance. You may notice improved posture, lubricated joints, better focus, and increased energy after doing yoga regularly.

We oxygenate our bodies when we do yoga. There's a practice in yoga called a sun salutation or a Sun Salute. The idea is that you do this exercise first thing in the morning with your body waking up and your cortisol levels bouncing up into their high ranges, getting your body moving and shaking off the sleep. Sun Salutation takes five to 10 minutes.

If you haven't done yoga before, be sure to go slowly at first and don't overdo it. Over time, you'll likely notice improvements to your strength and endurance.

BODYWEIGHT EXERCISE

You don't need to have a gym membership to take part in effective bodyweight exercise. Your body provides all the equipment you need for a great workout!

You can search the internet for great bodyweight exercises or follow simple workouts that have been done for decades – like pushups, pullups, jumping jacks, and lunges. The point of bodyweight exercise is to move your body in all directions and on all planes every day.

WHAT ABOUT INTENSITY?

The old-school way of exercising, which many people still do, is long, slow exercise at mild to moderate intensity. Think of a 60-minute aerobics class or 45 minutes on the treadmill, watching the TV. Or you may see someone at the gym doing 40 reps with a two-pound dumbbell.

The new and improved method of exercise is to perform short, fast bursts of high intensity or at least moderate-intensity activities. How does that look? Let's say you're on a treadmill, and instead of going at moderate intensity, you run as fast as you can sprint for 30 seconds, and then you slow down and walk for a minute. Then you sprint for another 30 seconds and then walk for a minute, and you continue this method for 15-20 minutes. You can also do this on a bike, in the pool, on a stair stepper, or on an elliptical machine. You could do this without any machines at all by running in place and kicking your knees up high. It doesn't matter how you do it, but the intensity should be as high as you can go. Try to achieve at least a moderate pace.

You can also do this high-intensity form of workout with weights. Instead of finding the weight you can lift 30 or 40 times, use the weight you can barely lift ten times. Max out the weight you're lifting and minimize the repetitions. If you do that, you'll burn those muscles out quicker, and you can move on to the next exercise.

The concept is to finish with your workout in 20 or 30 minutes, which is a win all around because most people are busy, and the time constraint is one of the main reasons people aren't working out.

When we do high intensity for short durations, our metabolism elevates for the next 24 hours. When we do low intensity for a short or long duration, our body burns calories while we're doing the exercise, but when we finish exercising, it stops. The net effect of a shorter period, higher intensity workout is more significant than long duration, mild intensity.

We all have to start somewhere. One person's high intensity won't be the same as somebody else's. Maybe going for a walk is intense for you right now, and that's okay. The more you do, the more your capacity increases, so your intensity can increase.

Pay attention to how your body feels. You will see amazing transformations in your strength, lean muscle mass, cardiovascular endurance, flexibility, mental health, and the rest of your physical health.

TAKE ACTION: IMPLEMENT MOVEMENT IN YOUR DAILY LIFE

THE FIRST SIX WEEKS (RESET): MOVEMENT AND FLEXIBILITY

As you begin to reset your body through the Simple Seven lifestyle, increase your movement and activity. Walk, do mild yoga, and stretch for the first six weeks as you reset your body. You don't need to participate in intense exercise at first.

THE NEXT FEW WEEKS (SUSTAIN): INCREASE INTENSITY

As you enter the "sustain" phase of the Simple Seven habits, you can ramp up the intensity of your workout. Begin incorporating some of the higher intensity exercises mentioned previously but take it at your own speed. You'll grow in strength and endurance as you continue to make these workouts a part of your daily routine.

A FEW MORE WEEKS AND BEYOND (MAINTENANCE): CONTINUE TO BUILD STRENGTH AND ENDURANCE

When you've fully implemented the Simple Seven strategies into your life, it's essential to maintain your new habits. You can continue to work out to build strength and endurance but remember that you're not trying to become a bodybuilder or an Olympic athlete. The goal is to build lean muscle, be able to move in a full range of motion without pain and maintain healthy movement for the rest of your life.

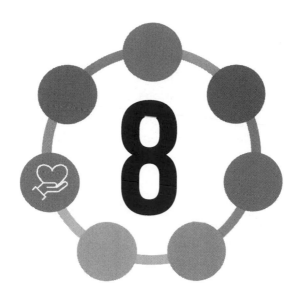

LOVE WELL

THE IMPORTANCE OF RELATIONSHIPS

As humans, our relationships with other people are vital to our mental and emotional well-being and survival. We have an inherent desire to be close to other people. Having supportive relationships, whether with a romantic partner, friends, and family members, can make for a healthier overall life.

When we feel loved and connected, we feel whole. Feeling loved and supported by a tribe is often directly related to our level of happiness.

Of course, relationships also have the power to make us miserable. Being in the wrong relationship or being surrounded by people who don't make us feel good or take advantage of us can feel awful and drain us emotionally.

Because relationships are so powerful, we have to learn how to cultivate fulfilling and healthy relationships. The basics of a healthy relationship tend to include the following:

- Listening to each other
- Communicating openly and without judgment
- Trust and respect for each other
- Remembering important details about each other's lives

We'll dive into some of the scientific benefits of being in a loving, healthy relationship.

LESS STRESS

Being in a committed relationship is linked to less production of cortisol, a stress hormone. This suggests that married or paired people are less responsive to psychological stress and that the social and emotional support that comes with having a partner can be a great way to combat stress.

GREATER SENSE OF PURPOSE

It's natural for humans to want to feel needed and part of something bigger. Many people strive to feel like they're doing something good for someone else and improving the world in some way. Being in a loving relationship, no matter what kind, can give a person a sense of well-being and purpose. It's possible that having a sense of purpose can add years to your life.

LONGER LIFE

Research also suggests that having healthy social relationships makes a more significant impact on avoiding early death. One study even suggests that a lack of social relationships affects health as much as smoking 15 cigarettes a day.[7]

---

[7] https://www.hrsa.gov/enews/past-issues/2019/january-17/loneliness-epidemic

THE 7 CORE RELATIONSHIPS

We believe there are seven core relationships. When these relationships continue to be cultivated and improved, they become beneficial and loving relationships that help your life be more fulfilling and happier.

RELATIONSHIP WITH SELF

Imagine being in a relationship with someone who said they loved you, but they always talked bad about you, pointed out your flaws regularly, told you were worthless, not good enough, or stupid. Now imagine you are stuck in this relationship for the rest of your life. How would that relationship feel? How would it affect your thoughts and feelings and ultimately your behavior?

Consider the relationship you have with yourself. Would you treat someone else the way you sometimes treat yourself? Would you speak to someone else the way you sometimes talk to yourself?

Here are some ideas to help you build a better relationship with yourself:

- **Invest in Yourself.** Spend time every day doing something you love.
- **Quiet the Inner Critic**. When your inner critic finds faults, remind yourself of how amazing you are by giving specific examples. (Inner critic, "You're so slow." Self-affirmation, "I always take the time to do things well."
- **Be Compassionate with Yourself.** When you make a mistake, don't beat yourself up. Act like you would if you were your own best friend by being kind, supportive, and forgiving.

RELATIONSHIP WITH A HIGHER POWER

A relationship with a higher power – God, Universe, nature, whatever that means for you – can generate meaning and purpose in your life.

This relationship helps us develop a deep, meaningful connection with something greater than ourselves. This relationship can promote a sense of comfort, trust, meaning, and purpose.

Religious affiliation is a powerful way to cultivate a spiritual life, but many people find their spiritual center outside of religion.

As you build a relationship with a higher power and develop spiritual connections, you will gain a deeper appreciation for yourself, others, and nature.

Here are a few ways to build a better relationship with your higher power:

- Spend time in nature
- Meditate
- Pray
- Get quiet and listen for guidance
- Tap into your intuition

RELATIONSHIP WITH PARENTS

Parent-child relationships go through various changes as the child grows from infancy through adulthood. Adulthood also has many different stages that can again change the relationship between the child and the parent.

A funny thing happens when you become an adult. You finally start to realize that your parents are real humans, flaws, and all. Navigating these family roles takes time, practice, and lots of communication.

Here are a few ways to build a better relationship with your parents:

- **Be Respectful.** Treat any differences with respect.
- **Take Responsibility for the Relationship.** Both parents and adult children hold responsibility for shaping, maintaining, and managing the relationship. That effort includes initiating contact, compromising, and negotiating, and finding mutually enjoyable ways to connect.

- **Be Compassionate.** Give your parents the same patience and understanding that you would give to anyone you care for. Try to view challenges as an opportunity for growth.

RELATIONSHIP WITH SPOUSE/PARTNER

Good relationships don't happen overnight. They take commitment, compromise, forgiveness, and most of all — effort.

Falling in love is the easy part. The challenge for couples is how to rekindle the fires of romance from time to time and cultivate the mature, trusting love that is the hallmark of a lasting relationship.

Generally, when you're happy in your relationship with your spouse, you tend to be more satisfied with your job, kids, social life, and everything else life throws your way. When you have someone that you love and trust to go through life with, even the difficult times seem more manageable.

Here are a few ways to build a better relationship with your partner or spouse:

- **Be Your Best.** Consciously offer your spouse your best self. Just like you took extra care to dress your best and act your best on your first date, try to be your best every day.
- **Talk.** Communication is key to keeping a relationship strong.
- **Say and Show "I Love You" Often.** Verbalizing love through compliments, words of appreciation, etc., speaks to those who need to hear love. Physical actions from touching to completing that "To-Do-List" speak to those who need to feel love through acts of kindness of physical connection.
- **Believe in Them.** Encourage and support your spouse in their goals and dreams.

RELATIONSHIP WITH CHILDREN

A child will rely on you for all their basic needs, both physical and emotional, when they're young. As a child grows, an engaged parent will teach self-reliance in both physical and emotional ways so that the child can eventually claim their autonomy from their parents.

Parents need to be willing to trust their child as they grow into an adult, trust them to forge their path, and learn their lessons by making their own mistakes. Of course, as a parent, we don't want to see our children suffer at any age but suffering through failure or disappointment also teaches resilience and valuable lessons that can also lead to great success and happiness.

Here are a few ideas to better connect with your children:

- **Show Your Love.** We need human touch and loving affection at every stage of our lives.
- **Show You're Interested in Them.** Learn about your child's interests. Participate in things they like to do and encourage them to explore the things they enjoy.
- **Show Them Your Weaknesses.** Let them see that you make mistakes, get angry, or experience failure. Then teach them how to try again, apologize, and manage their emotions.
- **Set Boundaries.** Young children and teens need structure and guidance to grow and learn about the world around them. Boundaries for adult children could include what level of privacy and involvement they seek and accept from parents, particularly in their career, relationships, lifestyle, and finance.

RELATIONSHIP TO COMMUNITY

Building and sustaining relationships is at the heart of a community. The strength of community lies in the power of the connections we have with each other. There is no telling what you can do with a strong connection of friends, colleagues, associates, allies, partners, and buddies around you.

The idea that we should treat our neighbors the way we would like to be treated is central to almost every religion. If you keep that in mind, you will most likely succeed in building relationships you can depend on.

Here are a few ways to build better relationships in your community:

- **Be Friendly and Make Connections.** A friendly word or smile can make someone's day. Try to find something in common: all of us want to have close connections with others.
- **Go Places and Do Things.** If you want to make friends, you have to go where the people are – like picnics, conferences, events, fundraisers, parties, playgrounds, bowling alleys, little league games, bake sales, etc.
- **Accept People.** Not everyone thinks or believes the same way as we do, but that shouldn't keep us from forming relationships with others. Often when we get to know people, our differences become strengths in the relationship because we can see so many other points of view or solutions to problems.

RELATIONSHIP TO RESOURCES

Our relationship with resources includes all non-human things. This is probably the biggest category of relationships that we have, but it is one that we may not think of as often. These types of relationships include our connection with the animal kingdom, objects, or the planet. Our relationship with resources may start with something large and break down to something smaller and smaller. For example, the large category of objects could break down smaller like this: our home, our furniture, our books, our dishes, our groceries, our linens, and clothes, and trinkets, etc.

These relationships are around us all the time, but we may not be paying attention to them. We may show love and respect to them, or we may show anger and resentment towards them. Consider that for a moment. Are there things in your life that you dislike and irritate you regularly?

Imagine you have a dishwasher, but it's broken. Every time you eat, you have to do dishes by hand, and every time you do that, you look at the broken dishwasher and have thoughts about it. Thoughts like, *"Why is that dumb thing still broken?"* or *"I really need to take time and get that fixed"*, and so on. Or you could also look at it and think something positive like, *"I'm so thankful that broke, now I get to spend time doing dishes every night with my spouse, and it's a great time for us to talk and connect"*.

Our relationship with our resources affects our lives and our human relationships.

Here are a few ways to build a better relationship with your resources:

- **Be Grateful.** Having gratitude for the things that we have helps us appreciate them more.
- **Take Care of Your Possessions**. Take care of the things you have just like you would take care of yourself or your children. They will last longer and serve their purpose for you better.
- **Do Your Part.** Investing in something helps us appreciate it and feel a sense of ownership. For example, we can take care of the earth by doing our part to be aware of natural resources and how we can protect and preserve them through our daily choices.

CULTIVATING HEALTHY RELATIONSHIPS

While no relationship is perfect and all relationships have their ups and downs, you never want to be stuck in a relationship that's doing more harm than good. Set realistic expectations for your relationships with others. You can't control other people's behavior, but you can be in charge of your own.

The following practices will help you cultivate healthy relationships and walk through the world with an attitude of calm warmth that remains steady, regardless of how others greet or treat you.

STAY TRUE TO WHO YOU ARE

It can be easy to compare ourselves to a friend with an infectious personality or a charismatic partner. While it's wonderful to appreciate someone for who they are, you should also embrace your unique gifts!

Remember, there's a reason people like you in the first place, so don't lose your distinctive qualities. Keep your own goals and growth in mind regardless of those you have relationships with.

Most importantly, love yourself first. The relationship you have with yourself should always be your top and most important relationship. Without a relationship with yourself, it is nearly impossible to form meaningful relationships with anyone else.

Just like other relationships in your life, take the time to get to know yourself, find out what makes you feel good, what makes you feel bad, and be curious as to why.

How you treat or feel about yourself will ultimately be how you project onto others. If we're harsh and self-critical with ourselves, we won't let anyone else off the hook either. If we grant ourselves love and acceptance, we open the door to treating others the same way.

PRACTICE EMPATHY

Empathy means to put yourself in someone else's shoes. Take a moment to think about how others might be feeling in their given situation and act respectfully and thoughtfully according to that situation.

Everyone is on their journey, and it can be hard sometimes to remember that something may affect another person entirely different than it would affect you. The enemy of empathy is self-centeredness, selfishness, or entitlement, so make strides to eliminate those tendencies from your relationships.

The most successful relationship dynamics are when each person involved in the relationship has a strong sense of empathy. If you want to develop a real sense of intimacy and closeness with another person, you must put yourself in their shoes. Empathy is the foundation and core of any successful relationship.

Remember this from Mary Lou Kownacki: "There isn't anyone you couldn't love once you've heard their story."

COMMUNICATION IS KEY

Constant communication doesn't mean that you're talking, texting, or calling each other nonstop. But remaining open to communication when there's confusion or a misunderstanding is crucial.

To simply shut down and avoid a problem will only make a relationship worse. Talk about issues when they come up.

You or your friend or partner may be the type who needs to take a step back before a discussion. It's fine to take time to cool off or think as long as you can discuss things shortly afterward.

BE HONEST, RELIABLE, AND CONSISTENT

One of the worst things you could do to sabotage any relationship is being dishonest. Nobody likes someone who doesn't follow through, doesn't follow through, or makes empty promises. Part of establishing a trusting relationship is showing up and doing what you say you're going to do. If you're unreliable in one aspect of your life, there's a good chance you're unreliable in other ways too. You can only get away with flaky behavior for so long before people stop putting up with it.

Keep in mind that a good foundation for any relationship is one built on trust.

SET BOUNDARIES

If you find yourself in a relationship with someone who has little empathy, is not thoughtful, or does not compromise, it is essential to set boundaries. Boundaries protect you from hurtful relationships and add distance between you and another person. Ultimately, if boundaries don't solve the problem, then you may want to consider ending the relationship entirely if possible.

There is no point in having relationships that make you feel bad, drain you, and leave you resentful.

Keep in mind that you can apply boundaries to any subject. If your friend keeps borrowing money from you, let them know you won't lend them more money until they pay the first amount back. If your partner wants to spend every waking moment with you but you need alone time, set that boundary. It's all about knowing what's best for you, what's best for them, and finding an agreement.

PRACTICE COMPASSION AND GENEROSITY

Generosity is more about being emotionally generous rather than just buying your friends and family gifts. When Tammie's grandmother died recently, some of her friends wrote thoughtful cards, which meant the world to her and made her feel lucky to have them in her life. Simply checking in with someone regularly to show you care is a sign of thoughtfulness and generosity.

Compassion is a way to show appreciation or thoughtfulness through words, gift-giving, verbal appreciation, or any kind gesture that lets someone know you are thinking of them and that you care for them.

Compassion also means not judging others harshly. Harsh judgement prevents you from relationships and prevents you from embracing humanity with all its many flaws. This doesn't mean that you shouldn't notice other people's bad behavior or your own, though.

There is a vast difference between observing and condemning. Judging is an act of distancing yourself from others. You can observe while remaining impartial and compassionate. Someone's behavior may result from their experiences in life, so we should use empathy when observing others' actions.

CREATE FAIRNESS AND RECIPROCITY

Of course, all the previous practices don't work unless everyone in the relationship is actively practicing them. You don't need to keep score of who's being a putting in the effort and pulling your meaning the relationship doesn't feel one-sided or uneven. All healthy relationships require a degree of compromise and fairness. People who consistently take from others and expect people to give and bend over backward for them without lifting a finger are people who don't have many friends or any friendships of real substance.

All positive and healthy relationships should stem from something beyond just selfish needs. People are more inclined to want to do nice things for you when they feel like you honestly like them and have an experience where you have been of service to them.

TAKE ACTION: GRATITUDE TO THE RESCUE

Just about every relationship can be improved if we have an increase of gratitude for the good things it provides. Expressing gratitude is a great way to change your mindset. A situation that may seem to be all-consuming, overwhelming, and difficult can become a source of hope and joy by introducing thoughts of gratitude.

This 5-minute gratitude exercise is a wonderful way to banish the overwhelm and bring more peace into your life.

To start, take out five pieces of paper and a pen. Write one of the following titles on each piece of paper:

- Physical
- Family

- Relationships
- Material Things
- Spiritual

Under each heading, write out the numbers 1-20. You'll write twenty things you're grateful for in each category, giving you a list of 100 in the end. At first, you may look blankly at the page. Just keep your pen on the paper and wait for the thoughts of gratitude to come. Eventually, your brain will cooperate, and you'll get a rush of thoughts that you may not be able to keep up with.

We'll define each category to help you get started.

PHYSICAL

In this section, focus on any physical attribute you are grateful for or something that you can physically do. For example: *I'm grateful for eyes that can see and the ability to read.*

FAMILY

You can list names in this section, but you can also create a list of things you do with your family. For example: *I am grateful for my grandma and holiday traditions.*

RELATIONSHIPS

Consider important relationships in your life and be sure to include people who aren't in your family. Keep in mind relationships with pets you love as well. For example: *I am grateful for my next-door neighbor. I'm grateful for my sweet dog who comforts me when I'm feeling sad.*

MATERIAL THINGS

Think of all those things you're happy you don't have to go through life without, the things we sometimes take for granted. For example: *I'm grateful for a working car.*

SPIRITUAL

List the things in your life that you can't physically see, but that are a crucial aspect of your life. For example: *I am grateful for my belief in God and my knowledge of the power of prayer.*

Keep this list for you're grateful for in each category. Keep this list for those moments when you feel the overwhelm creeping in, when life is darker than light, and when nothing seems to be going right.

When we've gone through tough times in our life, we read the lists we've created, and within just a few minutes, life seems a little brighter as gratitude abounds. Your list can help you change your perspective, even when you're still stuck in the same difficulties that brought you down.

Gratitude is powerful! It will serve to connect you back to your heart, your community, and your soul. Gratitude nourishes you in ways food cannot. Studies have shown that regularly expressing gratitude is associated with lowered blood pressure, reduced stress hormone levels, a healthier heart, increased kidney function, and an overall sense of increased energy and vitality. Not bad for a quick moment of thanks!

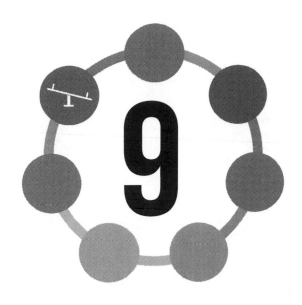

PLAY WELL

The last pillar of wellness hardly gets any attention these days, but it's much more important than people realize. You rarely see this item as a wellness tip or a way to contribute to overall well-being. We think this is a big oversight.

Most people consider diet, movement, sleep, a positive mental attitude, and loving relationships when improving wellness, so why have we added this last strategy? It's the key to joy and loving life, and it's what gives life a kind of sweetness. There's also scientific evidence that play is pivotal for our personal welfare.

THE GAME OF LIFE

In many ways, life is a game, it's an epic adventure, and unfortunately, most adults are just spectators. They're not really participating and diving into the amazing experience that lies ahead of them. Play is the root of creativity; it forms the basis for creative thoughts, great music, art, literature, and even the concepts of logic and problem-solving. This comes from the development of the ability to play in our youth and is essential for mental health. We often think the opposite of play is work, but really, the opposite of play is depression.

Play contextualizes memory. It lights up our brain as almost no other behavior does. Play is also transformative; it's the bedrock of socialization. It develops trust, interpersonal dynamics, and self-awareness.

FOUR TYPES OF PLAY

There are essentially four types of play. Physical play is "rough and tumble," such as physical game sports or movement-oriented play. Imaginative play is the kind where we play roles or make-believe. Constructive play is when we build or model things with our hands. There's also social play, which is engaging in activities with others, role-playing scenarios, or playing house. Some of these types of play may cross over; for example, social play could be role-playing, which uses some aspects of make-believe or suspends the laws of physics.

We'll dive into more detail to demonstrate why each of these types of play is so beneficial for a balanced life.

PHYSICAL PLAY

Physical play is the roughhousing your mom told you not to do inside, like chasing, tackling, and grappling. It's also sports, playing catch with your son, playing Frisbee with mom, or jumping on the trampoline. These are all physical movements that are either structured like a sport with clear rules or very unstructured, like skiing. Physical play is amazing because of its body component and the joy we feel when connected with our physical body movement.

IMAGINATIVE PLAY

When you think of imaginative play, you may think it's all about playing with dolls and action figures, but it's more than that! It's writing creatively, acting in theater, performing music, painting, and much more. Imaginative play allows us to let go of preconceptions and create a universe that behaves differently from real life. We can explore past preconceived limitations and let our minds wander. When we engage in this type of play, we can develop "out of the box" ideas.

If you feel like you aren't creative, the truth may be that you once were but have since lost it because you haven't engaged in imaginative play in so long. When we don't practice creativity, it can wither, but simple actions can bring it back, even in adulthood. Whether it's learning to draw or paint, making up a story, writing a poem (even if it's terrible), engaging in these activities is like working muscles that need to grow. The more you do it, the stronger you'll become.

CONSTRUCTIVE PLAY

Constructive play is beneficial for spatial awareness; we can manipulate physical objects like blocks, Legos or puzzle pieces or create something out of paper or cardboard. This is the process of coming up with ideas and trying to build something in an iterative process. If our ideas fail, we look at what we did wrong and try to figure out what we can do to make it better. It's where we take a concept, and we move it through to physical reality.

Constructive play is gratifying; it feeds our soul to create something out of nothing or create order out of chaos. The process of trial and error and observation and adjustment can help us develop the brain structure to solve complex problems in life.

When done in groups, this type also helps us develop our conflict resolution skills, interact with other people, and learn how to be vulnerable in a safe place.

SOCIAL PLAY

Social play is one of the most important types of recreation. This is a time when we interact with others, learn to follow the rules, share, respect others' differences, and so much more.

We've learned that when children engage in social play, they learn to communicate, collaborate, problem-solve, and so much more. If your child isn't getting enough social interaction with other children, you can often sense the issue and pinpoint the problem immediately.

Here's the thing: social play doesn't become unimportant when we're adults. It's just different. Social play for adults could mean taking part in a sport with a set of rules, like basketball or soccer, but you don't have to sign up for the local softball team to engage in social play. You could play volleyball with friends at the neighborhood park, build a snowman with your kids, play a board game with your family, and so much more.

HOW MUCH PLAY DO WE NEED?

Every type of play is invaluable for our overall wellness. Take a few seconds and think about your week. See if you can come up with a list of even a few things you did this past week that would fit in the description of play, then try to understand what type of play you engaged in.

As adults, we rarely engage in enough play because there's always so much work to do. We go from one thing to the next, and instead of "playing" when we're done working, we spend our time relaxing or simply being entertained. Watching a movie or bingeing on Netflix doesn't count as play—those activities don't engage the part of our brains that create.

So how much play do we need? Nobody really knows the answer to that, but we like to come up with ways to implement play into everyday life.

There's a concept called neoteny, which is the ability to retain youthful behaviors into adult life. Think of people you know who are old in years, but they've maintained a youthfulness and vibrancy in mind and behavior. They have a zest for life. These people have learned how to tap into this youthful creative play energy, which is instinctive when we're young, but most adults repress it.

Science is catching up to the seriousness of play and the fact that our brains need to stay young and vital. And here are a couple of ways to think about this. If the activity you're doing has a purpose above and beyond just the activity, it probably isn't play. For example, consider a professional basketball player. You can say they're playing the game of basketball, but the purpose of playing the game is different for a professional athlete than for someone playing a pickup game with friends on a Saturday. It's the athlete's vocation, their social platform. The athlete will still reap the physical benefits of playing basketball, but it isn't quite the same as engaging in play.

Many people have hobbies that are like their profession. Maybe someone who works as a computer coder has a hobby of coding games for fun. While this is still beneficial, it's not nearly as helpful as finding something separate from your work to develop a different part of who you are.

The goal is to infuse "play energy" into your life. It's not just something you do on Tuesday nights from 6:00-8:00 p.m. Think about ways you might be able to infuse more creativity, exploration, social dynamic, roleplay, and physicality in all the things you do. How can you approach your work with this mindset? What about your personal life and your relationships?

Infusing creative, expressive energy into your day could be the difference between being happy and enjoying your life versus being unhappy and depressed. You could do something as simple as creating a playlist of funny videos to watch on YouTube during lunch to get yourself into a more "playful" mode. Instead of spending your lunch hour trying to catch up on work, try shifting gears. Watch something that makes you laugh, walk around the block, draw, listen to music, or something else that gets you out of work mode for a bit.

See if this simple trick can help you to have a more youthful vibrancy throughout your day.

TAKE ACTION: MAKE YOUR PLAY LIST

You've heard of a music playlist; you probably have a few playing on repeat day after day. Similarly, you can create a "play" playlist to help implement this strategy into your life.

First, consider what activities you love to do. If you don't know, think about what you used to enjoy doing as a kid or a young adult. Try those activities again. List out three to five activities.

Next, try to think of a different type of play you could add to your life. If all the previously listed activities would be done by yourself, write out a few more things you enjoy doing that involve other people.

Finally, make it happen. If you need to schedule your recreation time, put it on your calendar. Sign up for a class or call a friend to invite them to join you. Try to implement all four types of play as often as you can.

You may have to do some mental work as you try to implement play into your daily routine. It might take some convincing yourself to feel that play is okay and even *healthy* for you. Play brings happiness and will significantly benefit your life! Try it out for yourself and see what happens.

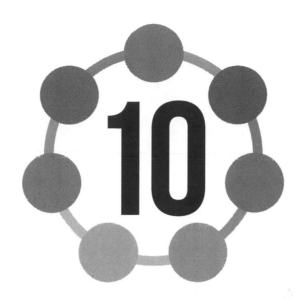

SUPPORT RESOURCES

When we set out to write this book, we consciously decided to do our best to keep our message simple and accurate. We wanted you to be able to finish a chapter quickly and have some actionable steps to take immediately. Above and beyond that, we wanted most of our recommendations to be as close to free as possible. We've seen so many people get lost in all the information available to them that they become confused, and a confused mind is a stuck mind. Here are a few additional tools to make sure that you never feel STUCK again!

GUIDES AND ACCOUNTABILY PARTNERS

It is so challenging for most of us to consistently engage in health promoting habits without some form of support and accountability. Experts in psychology have long known that having someone to be accountable to dramatically improves the likelihood of successfully implementing lifestyle changes.

We hope that as you begin to make positive shifts in your lifestyle that you will encourage those around you to make changes with you. Get creative with this. Try to start a small walking group. You could find some friends or family members to exchange healthy recipes with every week. How about offer to do a child-care swap with a friend so that you can each go out on a fun date with your significant other on a routine basis. In other words, create your own tribe of people who are all looking to make the most of their health. You'll find that creating these small communities are tools to supercharge your health.

The principles we've shared in this book provide the foundation for every recommendation we provide for our private clients. But what happens if these lifestyle changes aren't' enough to solve all of your health problems?

There are so many things that we can't control that can happen to us to cause our health to suffer, and in those situations, finding a health care provider who can help you identify the critical imbalances that are at the root of your condition is critical to real healing.

A NEW AND BETTER APPROACH

In the old days, you got sick, you went to the family doctor, he gave you some pills and you left. There was only one approach and one delivery system available. Western medicine (technically called Allopathic medicine) had a complete monopoly in the marketplace. Sure, there have always been people that preferred herbs and more natural methods but the promise of "better health from better drugs" was so appealing that those alternatives had virtually disappeared.

Well, times sure have changed. Now there are many different approaches available. While western medicine has certainly shown its tremendous value with urgent, lifesaving, heroic interventions, there are many critics who point out the shortcomings when it comes to managing chronic disease. It seems that model has mistakenly taught us that if we don't have symptoms, we are healthy. Well, science has proven that premise completely and woefully inadequate to really create the health we are all looking for. The new paradigm of understanding is that the symptom is often the last thing to show up in a process. In fact, the body can lose over 70% of its function before symptoms begin! The American health system is set up to do nothing until signs and symptoms are well under way in the body. This approach has caused America to slide to the bottom of the pile when it comes to the healthiest nations.

It's pretty clear to anyone who looks at the problem that we need a better approach. An approach to healthcare that involves the understanding of the underlying causes of dis-ease and dysfunction in the body, not just the symptom. That model is here, and it is called Functional Medicine.

Functional medicine physicians utilize advanced laboratory testing similar to conventional medicine but instead of using drugs to mask the symptoms, we attempt to restore balance to the body with nutrition, lifestyle, supplements and other safe and conservative approaches first. Medications are used sparingly if needed at all. This approach emphasizes true health creation instead of just disease prevention. It focuses on balancing systems not covering symptoms and it revolves around giving the patient the power to direct their own outcomes.

Right now there are thousands and thousands of physicians – medical doctors, osteopaths, chiropractors, naturopaths, nurses and more – who are leaving their old ways of practicing behind and embracing this new functional medicine model. They are saying goodbye to corporate medicine and getting back to the basics of personalized medicine. They are disrupting the status quo of healthcare and creating novel ways to try to bring the benefits of functional medicine to people at an affordable price.

WORK WITH US

FUNCTIONAL MEDICINE MEMBERSHIP

One exciting approach that is gaining a lot of traction in the marketplace among functional physicians and their patients is the "membership" approach. This model allows for each client to get a balance of personalized attention and time with their doctor and health coach but also leverages online technology to deliver a wide variety of education and coaching that can be delivered in a group setting.

If you are interested in learning more about how to engage with our team in our functional medicine membership program, please visit our website at www.duggarwellness.com

SIMPLE 7 LIFESTYLE RESET GROUP PROGRAM

In addition to our private, personalized membership program, we also have created a truly life changing 12-week group reset program that that is specifically geared to help you implement the Simple 7 Lifestyle and to reset your metabolism and shed unwanted body fat.

Our group reset clients typically lose well over 20 lbs. during this process but that just the tip of the iceberg. Jump over to www.simple7reset.com to learn more about the process and enroll in our next group.

ADDITIONAL READING

We hope that we've been successful in inspiring you to want to learn even more about any or all the Simple 7 Solutions. There are literally thousands of books available on these topics, so we thought we'd share our favorites to get you started.

CHAPTER 1 - THE BIG "WHY"

- *Unconventional Medicine* by Chris Kresser
- *Evolution of Medicine* by James Maskell

CHAPTER 2 - THE JOURNEY

- *The Conscious Creator* by Kris Krohn

CHAPTER 3 - THINK WELL

- *The Urban Monk* by Pedram Shojai

CHAPTER 4 - BREATHE WELL

- *Breath* by James Nestor
- *The Oxygen Advantage* by Patrick McKeown

CHAPTER 5 - SLEEP WELL

- *Sleep Smarter* by Shawn Stevenson

CHAPTER 6 - EAT WELL

- *Eat Smarter* by Shawn Stevenson
- *Food Fix* by Mark Hyman MD
- *The Paleo Cure* by Chris Kresser

CHAPTER 7 - MOVE WELL

- *Move Your DNA* by Katy Bowman

CHAPTER 8 - LOVE WELL

- *Love Yourself Like Your Life Depends On It* by Kamal Ravikant

CHAPTER 9 - PLAY WELL

- *Book of Play* by Michael Rosen